Current Controversies in Thoracic Surgery

Editor

MICHAEL LANUTI

THORACIC SURGERY CLINICS

www.thoracic.theclinics.com

Consulting Editor
M. BLAIR MARSHALL

August 2016 • Volume 26 • Number 3

ELSEVIER

1600 John F. Kennedy Boulevard • Suite 1800 • Philadelphia, Pennsylvania, 19103-2899

http://www.thoracic.theclinics.com

THORACIC SURGERY CLINICS Volume 26, Number 3
August 2016 ISSN 1547-4127, ISBN-13: 978-0-323-45991-4

Editor: John Vassallo (j.vassallo@elsevier.com)
Developmental Editor: Casey Jackson

Thoracic Surgery Clinics (ISSN 1547-4127) is published quarterly by Elsevier Inc., 360 Park Avenue South, New York, NY 10010-1710. Months of publication are February, May, August, and November. Business and editorial offices: 1600 John F. Kennedy Boulevard, Suite 1800, Philadelphia, PA 19103-2899. Periodicals postage paid at New York, NY, and additional mailing offices. Subscription prices are $355.00 per year (US individuals), $501.00 per year (US institutions), $100.00 per year (US Students), $435.00 per year (Canadian individuals), $648.00 per year (Canadian institutions), $225.00 per year (Canadian and international students), $465.00 per year (international individuals), and $648.00 per year (international institutions). Foreign air speed delivery is included in all Clinics' subscription prices. All prices are subject to change without notice. **POSTMASTER:** Send address changes to Thoracic Surgery Clinics, Elsevier Health Sciences Division, Subscription Customer Service, 3251 Riverport Lane, Maryland Heights, MO 63043. **Customer Service (orders, claims, online, change of address): Telephone: 1-800-654-2452 (U.S. and Canada); 314-447-8871 (outside U.S. and Canada). Fax: 314-447-8029. E-mail: journalscustomerservice-usa@elsevier.com (for print support); journalsonlinesupport-usa@elsevier.com (for online support).**

Reprints. For copies of 100 or more, of articles in this publication, please contact Commercial Rights Department, Elsevier Inc., 360 Park Avenue South, New York, NY 10010-1710. Tel: 212-633-3874; Fax: 212-633-3820; E-mail: reprints@elsevier.com.

Thoracic Surgery Clinics is covered in *MEDLINE/PubMed (Index Medicus), EMBASE/Excerpta Medica, Science Citation Index Expanded (SciSearch®), Journal Citation Reports/Science Edition,* and *Current Contents®/Clinical Medicine.*

Contributors

CONSULTING EDITOR

M. BLAIR MARSHALL, MD, FACS
Chief, Division of Thoracic Surgery, Associate
Professor, Department of Surgery,
Georgetown University Medical Center,
Georgetown University School of Medicine,
Washington, DC

EDITOR

MICHAEL LANUTI, MD, FACS
Associate Professor of Surgery, Harvard
Medical School; Director of Thoracic
Oncology, Division of Thoracic Surgery,
Massachusetts General Hospital, Boston,
Massachusetts

AUTHORS

USMAN AHMAD, MD
Division of Thoracic Surgery, Department of
Cardiothoracic Surgery, Heart and Vascular
Institute, Cleveland Clinic, Cleveland, Ohio

RAFAEL S. ANDRADE, MD
Associate Professor of Surgery; Chief, Section
of Thoracic and Foregut Surgery, Division of
Cardiothoracic Surgery, University of
Minnesota, Minneapolis, Minnesota

PAUL ARIDGIDES, MD
Assistant Professor, Department of Radiation
Oncology, SUNY Upstate Medical University,
Syracuse, New York

MARK F. BERRY, MD
Associate Professor, Department of
Cardiothoracic Surgery, Stanford University,
Stanford, California

JEFFREY BOGART, MD
Professor and Chairman, Department of
Radiation Oncology, SUNY Upstate Medical
University, Syracuse, New York

JESSICA S. DONINGTON, MD, MSCR
Associate Professor, Department of
Cardiothoracic Surgery, NYU School of
Medicine, New York, New York

RAJA M. FLORES, MD
Ames Professor of Cardiothoracic Surgery,
Chairman, Department of Thoracic Surgery,
Mount Sinai Health System, Icahn School of
Medicine, New York, New York

RICHARD K. FREEMAN, MD, MBA
Division of Thoracic and Cardiovascular
Surgery, St Vincent Hospital, Indianapolis,
Indiana

RAFAEL GARZA-CASTILLON Jr, MD
Thoracic Surgery Research Fellow, Section of
Thoracic and Foregut Surgery, Division of
Cardiothoracic Surgery, University of
Minnesota, Minneapolis, Minnesota

ERIN A. GILLASPIE, MD
Instructor in Surgery, Division of Thoracic
Surgery, Mayo Clinic, Rochester, Minnesota

OSWALDO GOMES Jr, MD
Department of Thoracic Surgery, University of São Paulo, São Paulo, Brazil

PRAVACHAN V.C. HEGDE, MD
Assistant Professor, Advanced Interventional Thoracic Endoscopy/Interventional Pulmonology, Division of Pulmonary and Critical Care Medicine, University of California San Francisco (UCSF), San Francisco, California

ARGENIS HERRERA, MD
Department of Surgery, St Vincent Hospital, Indianapolis, Indiana

JAMES HUANG, MD
Thoracic Service, Memorial Sloan Kettering Cancer Center, New York, New York

PAULO KAUFFMAN, PhD
Department of Vascular Surgery, University of São Paulo, São Paulo, Brazil

MICHAEL LANUTI, MD, FACS
Associate Professor of Surgery, Harvard Medical School; Director of Thoracic Oncology, Division of Thoracic Surgery, Massachusetts General Hospital, Boston, Massachusetts

MOISHE LIBERMAN, MD, PhD
Associate Professor, Division of Thoracic Surgery, Department of Surgery; Director, CHUM Endoscopic Tracheobronchial and Oesophageal Center (CETOC), Centre Hospitalier de l'Université de Montréal, University of Montreal, Montreal, Quebec, Canada

JOSE RIBAS MILANEZ DE CAMPOS, PhD
Department of Thoracic Surgery, University of São Paulo, São Paulo, Brazil

ASHOK MUNIAPPAN, MD
Department of Thoracic Surgery, Massachusetts General Hospital, Harvard Medical School, Boston, Massachusetts

EITAN PODGAETZ, MD, MPH
Assistant Professor of Surgery, Section of Thoracic and Foregut Surgery, Division of Cardiothoracic Surgery, University of Minnesota, Minneapolis, Minnesota

JOANNA SESTI, MD
Resident, Department of Cardiothoracic Surgery, NYU School of Medicine, New York, New York

SMITA SIHAG, MD
Department of Thoracic Surgery, Massachusetts General Hospital, Harvard Medical School, Boston, Massachusetts

DENNIS A. WIGLE, MD, PhD
Associate Professor and Chair, Division of Thoracic Surgery, Mayo Clinic, Rochester, Minnesota

ANDREA S. WOLF, MD, MPH
Assistant Professor, Department of Thoracic Surgery, Mount Sinai Health System, Icahn School of Medicine, New York, New York

NELSON WOLOSKER, PhD
Department of Vascular Surgery, University of São Paulo, São Paulo, Brazil

Contents

Preface: Managing Controversial Issues in Thoracic Surgery   ix

Michael Lanuti

**Mediastinal Staging: Endosonographic Ultrasound Lymph Node Biopsy or
Mediastinoscopy**   243

Pravachan V.C. Hegde and Moishe Liberman

Combined endosonographic lymph node biopsy techniques are a minimally invasive
alternative to surgical staging in non–small cell lung cancer and may be superior to
standard mediastinoscopy and surgical mediastinal staging techniques. Endosonography allows for the biopsy of lymph nodes and metastases unattainable with
standard mediastinoscopy. Standard cervical mediastinoscopy is an invasive procedure, which requires general anesthesia and is associated with higher risk,
cost, and major complication rates compared with minimally invasive endosonographic biopsy techniques. Combined endosonographic procedures are the new
gold standard in staging of non–small cell lung cancer when performed by an experienced operator.

**Sublobar Resection: Ongoing Controversy for Treatment for Stage I Non–Small Cell
Lung Cancer**   251

Joanna Sesti and Jessica S. Donington

Despite a prospective randomized trial that reported decreased locoregional recurrence for the intentional use of sublobar resection for stage IA non–small cell lung
cancer, it continues to be a point of considerable debate. Improved imaging techniques have introduced a large group of smaller and more indolent tumors than
what was studied 20 years ago by the Lung Cancer Study Group. Multiple single-
institution and population-based analyses suggest that sublobar resections may
have equivalent outcomes to lobectomy in well-selected patients with small
(<2 cm) resections, and in whom an adequate resection margin can be achieved.

Stereotactic Body Radiation Therapy for Stage I Non–Small Cell Lung Cancer   261

Paul Aridgides and Jeffrey Bogart

Stereotactic body radiation therapy (SBRT) has had a profound impact on the treatment paradigm for medically inoperable patients with stage I non–small cell lung
cancer. Local control and survival outcomes from prospective collaborative trials using SBRT have been highly favorable in this challenging patient population. Further
study in medically operable patients is ongoing; however, randomized trials to help
answer this question have terminated early because of poor accrual. Available prospective and retrospective data are discussed for the use of SBRT with regard to the
medically inoperable and operable patient populations, as well as considerations for
fractionation, dose, and toxicity.

Management of Stage IIIA (N2) Non–Small Cell Lung Cancer   271

Erin A. Gillaspie and Dennis A. Wigle

There is no consensus as to the optimal management of IIIA (N2) non–small cell lung
cancer, nor for the role of surgery in treating this disease stage. Clinical trial evidence

struggles to keep up with technology advancement and the evolution of expert opinion. Despite advances in chemotherapeutic regimens, methods of delivery for radiation, and less invasive surgical techniques, survival for patients with stage IIIA-N2 malignancies remains poor. Further developments in both will stimulate and maintain controversy in the field for years to come.

Surgical Management of Oligometastatic Non–Small Cell Lung Cancer   287
Michael Lanuti

Patients harboring stage IV non-small cell lung cancer represent a heterogeneous population with limited life expectancy. Targeted chemotherapy and immunotherapy have improved median survival for a minority of patients. A subset of patients with solitary foci of metastatic disease appears to have improved survival compared to others with stage IV NSCLC. The role of aggressive local control with curative intent for all disease sites in synchronous oligometastatic disease lacks randomized data; however, published retrospective series from single institutions suggest improved survival in highly selected patients (11–30%, 5-year survival) with low morbidity and mortality <2%.

The Role of Induction Therapy for Esophageal Cancer   295
Mark F. Berry

Survival of esophageal cancer generally is poor but has been improving. Induction chemoradiation is recommended before esophagectomy for locally advanced squamous cell carcinoma. Both induction chemotherapy and induction chemoradiation are found to be beneficial for locally advanced adenocarcinoma. Although a clear advantage of either strategy has not yet been demonstrated, consensus-based guidelines recommend induction chemoradiation for locally advanced adenocarcinoma.

The Evolution and Current Utility of Esophageal Stent Placement for the Treatment of Acute Esophageal Perforation   305
Argenis Herrera and Richard K. Freeman

Esophageal stent placement was used primarily for the treatment of malignant strictures until the development of a new generation of biomaterials allowed the production of easily removable, occlusive stents in 2001. Since then, thoracic surgeons have gained experience using esophageal stents for the treatment of acute esophageal perforation. As part of a hybrid treatment strategy, including surgical drainage of infected spaces, enteral nutrition, and aggressive supportive care, esophageal stent placement has produced results that can exceed those of traditional surgical repair. This review summarizes the evolution of esophageal stent use for acute perforation and provides evidence-based recommendations for the technique.

Lymph Node Dissection and Pulmonary Metastasectomy   315
Smita Sihag and Ashok Muniappan

Unexpected lymph node involvement is observed in approximately 20% of all patients undergoing pulmonary metastasectomy. Lymph node metastasis is often associated with decreased survival in patients with pulmonary metastases. The incidence of lymph node involvement is related to a variety of patient and tumor variables. This article reviews the indications and role for lymph node assessment at pulmonary metastasectomy.

Induction Therapy for Thymoma 325

Usman Ahmad and James Huang

> Thymomas are uncommon tumors that can present as locally advanced tumors in approximately 30% of the patients. Stage and complete resection are the strongest prognostic factors. For locally advanced tumors, induction treatment may improve the ability to achieve a complete resection. Combination treatment with cisplatin, doxorubicin, and cyclophosphamide is the most commonly used induction regimen. Similar rates of resectability are noted with the use of induction chemotherapy and chemoradiation therapy; however, more tumor necrosis is noted with the addition of radiation.

Best Approach and Benefit of Plication for Paralyzed Diaphragm 333

Eitan Podgaetz, Rafael Garza-Castillon Jr, and Rafael S. Andrade

> Diaphragmatic eventration and diaphragmatic paralysis are 2 entities with different etiology and pathology, and are often clinically indistinguishable. When symptomatic, their treatment is the same, with the objective to reduce the dysfunctional cephalad excursion of the diaphragm during inspiration. This can be achieved with diaphragmatic plication through the thorax or the abdomen with either open or minimally invasive techniques. We prefer the laparoscopic approach, due to its easy access to the diaphragm and to avoid pain associated with intercostal incisions and instrument use. Short-term and long-term results are excellent with this technique.

Video-Assisted Thoracic Sympathectomy for Hyperhidrosis 347

Jose Ribas Milanez de Campos, Paulo Kauffman, Oswaldo Gomes Jr, and Nelson Wolosker

> By the 1980s, endoscopy was in use by some groups in sympathetic denervation of the upper limbs with vascular indications. Low morbidity, cosmetic results, reduction in the incidence of Horner syndrome, and the shortened time in hospital made video-assisted thoracic sympathectomy (VATS) better accepted by those undergoing treatment for hyperhidrosis. Over the last 25 years, this surgical procedure has become routine in the treatment of hyperhidrosis, leading to a significant increase in the number of papers on the subject in the literature.

Current Treatment of Mesothelioma: Extrapleural Pneumonectomy Versus Pleurectomy/Decortication 359

Andrea S. Wolf and Raja M. Flores

> The role of surgical resection in malignant pleural mesothelioma (MPM) is based on the principle of macroscopic resection of a solid tumor with adjuvant therapy to treat micrometastatic disease. Extrapleural pneumonectomy (EPP) and pleurectomy decortication (P/D) have been developed in this context. Cancer-directed surgery for MPM is associated with a 5-year survival rate of 15%. Evidence indicates that P/D is better tolerated by patients and suggests survival is no worse when compared with EPP. Although EPP is still performed in highly selected cases, the authors advocate radical P/D whenever possible for patients with MPM.

Index 377

THORACIC SURGERY CLINICS

FORTHCOMING ISSUES

November 2016
Hyperhidrosis
Peter B. Licht, *Editor*

February 2017
Clinical Management of Chest Tubes
Pier Luigi Filosso, *Editor*

May 2017
The Chest Wall
Henning Gaissert, *Editor*

RECENT ISSUES

May 2016
Innovations in Thoracic Surgery
Kazuhiro Yasufuku, *Editor*

February 2016
Pulmonary Metastasectomy
Mark W. Onaitis and
Thomas A. D'Amico, *Editors*

November 2015
**Prevention and Management of
Postoperative Complications**
John D. Mitchell, *Editor*

RELATED INTEREST

Surgical Oncology Clinics, Volume 25, Issue 3 (July 2016)
Lung Cancer
Mark J. Krasna, *Editor*
Available at: www.surgonc.theclinics.com

THE CLINICS ARE AVAILABLE ONLINE!
Access your subscription at:
www.theclinics.com

Preface
Managing Controversial Issues in Thoracic Surgery

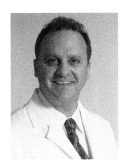

Michael Lanuti, MD, FACS
Editor

This issue of *Thoracic Surgery Clinics* depicts the contemporary controversies around the management of both benign and malignant conditions in Thoracic Surgery. The discussions are very relevant to the daily practice of surgeons and provide an organized summary and interpretation of the latest published literature relevant to each topic. Many issues in our field remain controversial by virtue of a paucity of prospective, randomized clinical trials, which assess the latest advance in treatments (ie, stereotactic body radiation therapy for stage I non–small cell lung cancer [NSCLC], approach to oligometastatic NSCLC, multimodality treatment of stage IIIA NSCLC, management of locally advanced thymoma, efficacy of lymph node dissection in pulmonary metastectomy) or surgical innovations (endobronchial ultrasound in staging lung cancer, benefit of surgical plication of a paralyzed diaphragm, stenting esophageal perforations, or efficacy of sympathectomy for focal hyperhidrosis). These areas of controversy are not necessarily comprehensive reviews of the literature, but a working prospective on each issue that may provide additional clarity. I thank the contributing authors for their valuable time and expertise in summarizing these specific areas of controversy.

Michael Lanuti, MD, FACS
Associate Professor of Surgery
Harvard Medical School
Director of Thoracic Oncology
Division of Thoracic Surgery
Massachusetts General Hospital
55 Fruit Street, Blake 1570
Boston, MA 02114, USA

E-mail address:
mlanuti@mgh.harvard.edu

Thorac Surg Clin 26 (2016) ix
http://dx.doi.org/10.1016/j.thorsurg.2016.05.001
1547-4127/16/$ – see front matter © 2016 Published by Elsevier Inc.

Mediastinal Staging
Endosonographic Ultrasound Lymph Node Biopsy or Mediastinoscopy

Pravachan V.C. Hegde, MD[a],*, Moishe Liberman, MD, PhD[b]

KEYWORDS

- Mediastinoscopy • Endoscopic lung cancer staging • Combined EBUS-EUS • Lung cancer staging
- Endobronchial ultrasound (EBUS) • Endoscopic ultrasound (EUS)
- Endosonographic lung cancer staging

KEY POINTS

- Staging is indicated in all central tumors, peripheral tumors larger than 3 cm, computed tomography (CT) scan showing lymph nodes larger than 1 cm, N1 lymph node involvement on PET, and PET positivity (standardized uptake value [SUV] >2) even if lymph node size less than 1 cm.
- Certain situations mandate nodal staging in the setting of normal PET and CT scans in the mediastinum. These situations include; central tumors, positive N1 nodes on CT and if there is low fludeoxyglucose uptake (SUV <2) in the primary tumor.
- The negative predictive value of combined endobronchial ultrasound (EBUS)–endoscopic ultrasound (EUS) is higher compared with standard mediastinoscopy. In comparison with conventional mediastinoscopy, endosonographic staging is less invasive and is carried out as an outpatient day case under conscious sedation, with considerable cost savings and also well tolerated by patients.
- Conventional mediastinoscopy is no longer the gold standard, and it is the end of the era of a traditional gold standard test.
- When compared with traditional mediastinoscopy, the ability of the combined EBUS-EUS technique to sample multiple stations and distant metastases, including structures below the diaphragm, with higher sensitivity and negative predictive value makes it a new gold standard in staging non–small cell lung cancer when performed by an experienced operator.

INTRODUCTION

Precise staging of the mediastinum is vital in determining the appropriate treatment plan in patients with potentially operable non–small cell lung cancer. Testing with invasive, minimally invasive, or noninvasive tests can prevent surgery and pulmonary resection in patients with advanced, benign, or medically treated diseases. Computed tomography (CT) and PET-CT scans have improved radiological staging of lung cancer; however, these techniques cannot provide definitive tissue diagnosis and are associated with high false-positive rates and low sensitivities and specificities.[1–9] Therefore, it is very important to confirm

The authors report no commercial or financial conflicts of interest. There are no funding sources.
[a] Fresno Medical Education Program, Advanced Interventional Thoracic Endoscopy/Interventional Pulmonology, Division of Pulmonary & Critical Care Medicine, University of California San Francisco (UCSF), 2335 East Kashian Lane, Suite 260, Fresno, CA 93701, USA; [b] Division of Thoracic Surgery, Department of Surgery, CHUM Endoscopic Tracheobronchial and Oesophageal Center (CETOC), Centre Hospitalier de l'Université de Montréal, University of Montreal, 1560 Sherbrooke Street East, 8e CD, Pavillon Lachapelle, Suite D-8051, Montreal, Quebec H2L 4M1, Canada
* Corresponding author.
E-mail address: phegde@fresno.ucsf.edu

Thorac Surg Clin 26 (2016) 243–249
http://dx.doi.org/10.1016/j.thorsurg.2016.04.005
1547-4127/16/$ – see front matter © 2016 Elsevier Inc. All rights reserved.

thoracic.theclinics.com

a positive N2 or N3 lymph node on PET-CT scan with a definitive tissue diagnosis. In this article, the authors discuss the current controversy between surgical and endosonographic mediastinal staging and the reasons why the authors think combined endosonographic lymph node staging should be the new gold standard in staging non–small cell lung cancer.

WHY DO WE STAGE IN NON–SMALL CELL LUNG CANCER?

Stage dictates therapy in non–small cell lung cancer. Staging helps to identify N2/N3 lymph nodes and distant metastases and thereby prevents futile thoracotomies/video-assisted thoracoscopic surgery (VATS). Staging is also important in certain circumstances in order to identify N1 lymph node metastases in candidates with poor lung function before planning stereotactic radiosurgery or sublobar resection.

IN WHOM DO WE INVASIVELY STAGE THE MEDIASTINUM IN NON–SMALL CELL LUNG CANCER?

According to the current guidelines from the American College of Chest Physicians (ACCP), National Comprehensive Cancer Network, European Respiratory Society, and European Society of Thoracic Surgeons (ESTS), staging is indicated in all central tumors, peripheral tumors larger than 3 cm, CT scans showing lymph nodes larger than 1 cm, N1 lymph node involvement on PET, and PET positivity (standardized uptake value [SUV] >2) even if lymph node size is less than 1 cm. Certain situations mandate nodal staging in the setting of normal PET and CT scans in the mediastinum. These situations include central tumors, positive N1 nodes on CT, and if there is low fludeoxyglucose (FDG) uptake (SUV <2) in the primary tumor.

WHO DOES NOT NEED INVASIVE MEDIASTINAL STAGING IN NON–SMALL CELL LUNG CANCER?

Patients with peripheral tumor size less than 3 cm (T1a-T1b) with no lymph node involvement on CT and no or low SUV (<2) uptake of the lymph node on PET scan do not need invasive mediastinal staging.

WHAT IS AN IDEAL GOLD STANDARD TEST IN STAGING LUNG CANCER?

The test should be able to get tissue diagnosis from most lymph nodes and metastases. It should

have a high sensitivity, specificity, accuracy, and negative predictive value. The complication rate should be low. It should be safe and cost-effective.

The traditional gold standard test in mediastinal lymph node staging has been cervical mediastinoscopy. The authors now discuss the reasons as to why mediastinoscopy may no longer be the gold standard for invasive mediastinal staging and why it is time to put an end to the era of a traditional gold standard surgical procedure.

ENDOSONOGRAPHIC ULTRASOUND (COMBINED ENDOBRONCHIAL ULTRASOUND–ENDOSCOPIC ULTRASOUND), LYMPH NODE BIOPSY, OR MEDIASTINOSCOPY?
Lymph Node Access, Sensitivity, Accuracy, and Negative Predictive Value

Standard mediastinoscopy allows access to stations 2R, 2L, 4R, 4L, 7, 10R, and 10L (**Fig. 1, Table 1**). Access to posterior and inferior mediastinum is limited. Sensitivity of mediastinoscopy has been reported to be between 79% and 93% with a false-negative rate of 8% to 11%.[10–12] Standard mediastinoscopy can access the paratracheal and subcarinal lymph node stations but not the paraesophageal, inferior pulmonary ligament,[8,9] and aortopulmonary (AP) window and para-aortic[5,6] lymph node stations. In addition, the lower aspect of the subcarinal

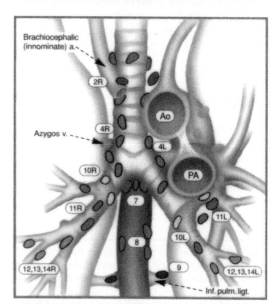

Fig. 1. Lymph node stations. PA, pulmonary artery; AO, aorta; Inf.pulm.ligt, inferior pulmonary ligament; a, artery; v, vein. (*Adapted from* Mountain CF, Dresler CM. Regional lymph node classification for lung cancer staging. Chest 1997;111:1718–1723. Copyright © 1996 Mountain and Dresler.)

Table 1
Lymph node accessibility with different procedural techniques

	EBUS	EUS	CM	AM	VATS
1: Highest mediastinal	✔	—	✔	—	—
2R: Upper paratracheal right	✓	✔	✔	—	✔
2L: Upper paratracheal left	✓	✓	✔	—	✔
3A: Prevascular	—	—	—	—	✔
3P: Retrotracheal	✔	✓	—	—	✔
4R: Lower paratracheal right	✓	—	✔	—	✔
4L: Lower paratracheal left	✓	✓	✔	—	✔
5: Subaortic (AP window)	—	✓	—	✔	✔
6: Para-aortic	—	NEW	—	✓	✓
7: Subcarinal	✓	✓	✔	—	✔
8: Paraesophageal	—	✓	—	—	✔
9: Pulmonary ligament	—	✓	—	—	✔
10: Hilar	✓	—	✔	—	✔
11: Interlobar	✓	—	—	—	✔

☑ indicates best initial diagnostic technique based on the anatomy of stations.
Abbreviations: AM, anterior mediastinotomy; CM, cervical mediastinoscopy; EBUS, endobronchial ultrasound; EUS, endoscopic ultrasound.
Data from Hegde P, Liberman M. Echo-endoscopic lymph node staging in lung cancer: an endoscopic alternative. Expert Rev Anticancer Ther 2015;15(9):1063–73; with permission.

station is sometimes inaccessible via standard mediastinoscopy. Interestingly, most of the N2 nodes missed by mediastinoscopy tend to be in those latter stations.[11,12]

Endobronchial ultrasound-guided transbronchial needle aspiration (EBUS-TBNA) allows access to stations 1, 2R, 2L, 3P, 4R, 4L, 7, 10R, 10L, 11R, 11L, 12R, and 12L. Occasionally, the 3A lymph node station can be reached by EBUS when the nodes are large enough. The sensitivity, specificity, negative predictive value, and accuracy of EBUS-TBNA are 93%, 100%, 91%, and 100%, respectively.[13–20] EBUS-TBNA is a minimally invasive technique to detect unsuspected nodal metastases in a radiologically normal mediastinum as well.[21,22] The sensitivity, specificity, negative predictive value, and diagnostic accuracy of EBUS-TBNA in a radiologically normal mediastinum are 93%, 100%, 87%, and 88%, respectively. In addition, EBUS is very helpful in detecting unsuspected nodal disease in medically inoperable patients being planned for stereotactic radiosurgery.[23]

Endoscopic ultrasound-guided fine-needle aspiration (EUS-FNA) allows access to stations 2R, 2L, 3P, 4L, 5, 7, 8, 9, celiac axis, left lobe of the liver, and left adrenal gland. The right adrenal gland can also be reached with a transduodenal approach. The 4R lymph node station can also be reached by EUS when the nodes are large enough (typically >2 cm). EUS is extremely helpful in reaching inferior mediastinum and structures below the diaphragm. There are new techniques to reach the para-aortic (station No. 6, **Fig. 2**) lymph nodes using EUS.[24,25] The sensitivity, specificity, positive predictive value, and negative predictive value of EUS-FNA are 92%, 100%, 100%, and 80%, respectively.[26] The sensitivity of EUS-FNA in a radiologically normal mediastinum is approximately 58%.[27] Adding EUS to EBUS is of benefit in complete endosonographic staging of the mediastinum.

Combined EBUS-EUS allows for greater evaluation of lymph node stations compared with a single technique alone, and the two techniques are complementary.[28–31] A prospective trial of 166 patients comparing combined EBUS-EUS and mediastinoscopy with final pathology results of lymph node sampling at pulmonary resection showed that EBUS-EUS was diagnostic for N2/N3/M1 disease in 14% of patients in whom standard mediastinoscopy findings were negative and thereby preventing futile thoracotomy.[31] The sensitivity, specificity, negative predictive value, and diagnostic accuracy of combined EBUS-EUS were 91%, 100%, 96%, and 97%, respectively (**Tables 2 and 3**). Endosonography has been reported to be more sensitive compared with surgical staging in detecting N2/N3 lymph nodal disease.[32] Studies comparing combined EBUS-EUS and transcervical extended mediastinal lymphadenectomy for negative results have concluded that in a

A

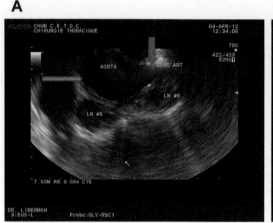

B

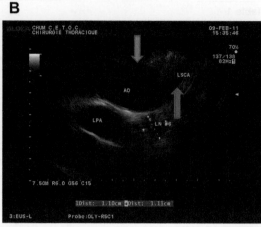

Fig. 2. (*A*) The aortic arch (*blue arrow*) with the left subclavian artery (*red arrow*) seen with EUS. Lymph nodes (LNs) 5 and 6 seen lateral (bottom of the screen) to the vessels. (*B*) LN station 6 lateral to the aortic arch (*blue arrow*) and the left subclavian artery (*red arrow*). The left pulmonary artery (LPA) is also seen. L SC ART, left subclavian artery; AO, aorta; LSCA, left subclavian artery.

radiologically normal mediastinum, if the results of EBUS-EUS are negative, then a surgical exploration of mediastinum can be omitted.[33] The authors do not recommend surgical staging even in an untreated FDG-avid lymph node if adequate lymphoid tissue was present in the specimen on combined EBUS-EUS FNA.

In addition, adding EUS to EBUS covers almost all the lymph node stations in the mediastinum and the commonly involved metastatic structures below the diaphragm. The sensitivity of endosonography increases with the addition of EUS to EBUS not only because of better visualization of inferior mediastinal nodes but also better visualization of station 4L and 7 lymph nodes and, in selected patients, the ability to access AP window lymph nodes. The sensitivity and negative predictive value of combined EBUS-EUS increases to 93% and 96% from 72% and 88% compared with EBUS alone. In the Assessment of Surgical sTaging vs Endoscopic Ultrasound in Lung Cancer: a

Randomized Clinical Trial (ASTER), the sensitivity of the endosonographic group was significantly higher (94%) than the surgical staging arm (79%). There were significantly fewer futile thoracotomies reported in the endosonographic group (7%) compared with the surgical staging arm (18%).[34]

Complication Rate

The complication rate of mediastinoscopy is significantly higher compared with minimally invasive endosonography techniques. The complication rate of mediastinoscopy is approximately 2%. Some of these complications are major, including recurrent laryngeal nerve palsy (0.05%), hemorrhage (0.32%), and tracheal injury (0.09%). Mortality has been reported to occur in 0.08% of patients related to pulmonary artery injury.[35] Although rare, when complications occur, they can be catastrophic. The complication rate of endosonographic biopsy techniques is approximately

Table 2
Endosonography versus standard cervical mediastinoscopy

	Sensitivity (%)	NPV (%)	Accuracy (%)
EBUS	72	88	91
EUS	62	85	88
EBUS + EUS	91	96	97

Abbreviation: NPV, negative predictive value.
Data from Liberman M, Sampalis J, Duranceau A, et al. Endosonographic mediastinal lymph node staging of lung cancer. Chest 2014;146(2):389–97.

Table 3
Mediastinal staging versus surgery

	NPV (%)	Accuracy (%)
EBUS	90	90
EUS	90	89
EBUS + EUS	92	91
Std CM	89	89

Abbreviations: NPV, negative predictive value; Std CM, standard cervical mediastinoscopy.
Data from Liberman M, Sampalis J, Duranceau A, et al. Endosonographic mediastinal lymph node staging of lung cancer. Chest 2014;146(2):389–97.

0.05%.[36] These complications include mediastinitis, airway injury, sepsis, pneumothorax, esophageal perforation, and mediastinal hematoma. No mortality has been reported in the literature.[37,38] The risk of infection is higher in cystic lesions and sarcoidosis.

Cost

The overall cost of mediastinoscopy is approximately $12,000, and the cost of EBUS-EUS done as a combined procedure in endoscopy unit under moderate sedation is approximately $4000. The cost of pulmonary resection is approximately $22,000.[39] There is no doubt that combined EBUS-EUS is more cost-effective than mediastinoscopy.

Restaging After Neoadjuvant Chemoradiation

There is a lack of evidence defining the role of endosonography and mediastinoscopy for restaging of the mediastinum after treatment in single station, nonbulky N2 node positive non–small cell lung cancer. The sensitivity of endosonography is significantly lower at 67% in this setting because of necrosis and fibrosis of the node due to chemotherapy.[40,41] Not many surgeons are comfortable doing a repeat mediastinoscopy for restaging purposes. The ACCP's guidelines comment that a repeat mediastinoscopy is safe and feasible; however, sensitivity is limited to about 70% to 82%. The ESTS emphasizes that a negative EBUS for restaging after neoadjuvant chemoradiation should be confirmed by invasive surgical mediastinal staging. It may be best to use endosonography as the initial staging modality and reserve surgical staging for restaging after neoadjuvant treatment in this particular situation, assuming that pulmonary resection is planned after neoadjuvant chemoradiation.

Aortopulmonary Window Lymph Nodes

In addition, AP window lymph nodes and para-aortic lymph nodes are not accessible by standard mediastinoscopy. The surgical modalities that can access these nodes are the Chamberlain procedure (left anterior mediastinotomy), extended cervical mediastinoscopy, and VATS. EUS can be helpful in selected cases to access AP window and para-aortic lymph nodes; however, this is an advanced technique not available in all centers.[24,25] If experienced operators are available, then EUS should be the first staging modality in accessing AP window and para-aortic lymph nodes particularly for left upper lobe lung cancers given the predilection of left upper lobe cancers to metastasize to these lymph nodes. If EUS is unsuccessful in providing adequate lymphocytes,

then alternative surgical modality should be considered for staging before pulmonary resection in this particular situation.

SUMMARY

In the authors' institution, combined EBUS-EUS staging for lung cancer has been performed routinely since 2009 in appropriately selected patients. Their results show a sensitivity of 91% and a negative predictive value of 96%.[31] Similar results have been reported by other centers in other studies looking at combined endosonographic lymph node staging with EBUS-EUS.[28–30] The negative predictive value of combined EBUS-EUS is higher than standard surgical mediastinoscopy.

Compared with conventional mediastinoscopy, endosonographic staging is less invasive and can be performed as an outpatient procedure under conscious sedation with considerable cost savings. The convenience of EBUS-EUS makes it an ideal staging test. It is fast, accurate, associated with a high negative predictive value, and well tolerated by patients. General anesthesia is not required. Multiple lymph node stations and the structures under the diaphragm can be sampled. It involves real-time imaging without radiation exposure. The equipment is portable. The overall procedure is cheap, safe, and provides a tissue diagnosis.

Similar to any operator-dependent procedure, there is variability in how effectively a staging procedure is actually performed. Every center has to look at their own yield and negative predictive value of any staging procedure as the experience and skill varies with the training of the operator. Endosonographic techniques were not invented to replace mediastinoscopy. The two techniques should not be considered competitive but should complement each other. The surgeon should choose the best minimally invasive approach for mediastinal staging depending on available resources. The relative simplicity, lower cost, and excellent sensitivity and negative predictive value of endosonographic techniques make it an attractive alternative to mediastinoscopy. Endosonography should be considered the new gold standard in invasive mediastinal staging of lung cancer. In addition, endoscopic staging can be repeated as necessary without increased morbidity.

REFERENCES

1. De Wever W, Ceyssens S, Mortelmans L, et al. Additional value of PET-CT in the staging of lung cancer: comparison with CT alone, PET alone and visual correlation of PET and CT. Eur Radiol 2007;17(1):23–32.

2. Silvestri GA, Gould MK, Margolis ML. American College of Chest Physicians. Non-invasive staging of nonsmall cell lung cancer: ACCP evidenced based clinical practice guidelines (2nd edition). Chest 2007;132(3):178S–201S.

3. Dales RE, Stark RM, Raman S. Computed tomography to stage lung cancer. Approaching a controversy using meta-analysis. Am Rev Respir Dis 1990;141(5.1):1096–101.

4. Lardinois D, Weder W, Hany TF. Staging of non-small-cell lung cancer with integrated positron-emission tomography and computed tomography. N Engl J Med 2003;348(25):2500–7.

5. Cerfolio RJ, Bryant AS, Ojha B, et al. Improving the inaccuracies of clinical staging of patients with NSCLC: a prospective trial. Ann Thorac Surg 2005; 80(4):1207–13.

6. McLoud TC, Bourgouin PM, Greenberg RW. Bronchogenic carcinoma: analysis of staging in the mediastinum with CT by correlative lymph node mapping and sampling. Radiology 1992;182(2): 319–23.

7. Tournoy KG, Maddens S, Gosselin R, et al. Integrated FDG-PET/CT does not make invasive staging of the intrathoracic lymph nodes in non-small cell lung cancer redundant: a prospective study. Thorax 2007;62(8):696–701.

8. Toloza EM, Harpole L, McCrory DC. Noninvasive staging of non-small cell lung cancer: a review of the current evidence. Chest 2003;123(1):137S–46S.

9. Silvestri GA, Hoffman B, Reed CE. Choosing between CT, positron emission tomography, endoscopic ultrasound with fine-needle aspiration, transbronchial needle aspiration, thoracoscopy, mediastinoscopy, and mediastinotomy for staging lung cancer. Chest 2003;123(2):333–5.

10. Detterbeck FC, Jantz MA, Wallace M, et al. American College of Chest Physicians. Invasive mediastinal staging of lung cancer: ACCP evidence-based clinical practice guidelines (2nd edition). Chest 2007; 132(Suppl 3):202S–20S.

11. Hammoud ZT, Anderson RC, Meyers BF, et al. The current role of mediastinoscopy in the evaluation of thoracic disease. J Thorac Cardiovasc Surg 1999; 118(5):894–9.

12. Lemaire A, Nikolic I, Petersen T, et al. Nine-year single center experience with cervical mediastinoscopy: complications and false negative rate. Ann Thorac Surg 2006;82(4):1185–9 [discussion: 1189–90].

13. Gu P, Zhao YZ, Jiang LY, et al. Endobronchial ultrasound-guided transbronchial needle aspiration for staging of lung cancer: a systematic review and meta-analysis. Eur J Cancer 2009;45(8): 1389–96.

14. Yasufuku K, Pierre A, Darling G, et al. A prospective controlled trial of endobronchial ultrasound-guided transbronchial needle aspiration compared with mediastinoscopy for mediastinal lymph node staging of lung cancer. J Thorac Cardiovasc Surg 2011;142(6): 1393–400.

15. Yasufuku K, Chiyo M, Sekine Y, et al. Real-time endobronchial ultrasound-guided transbronchial needle aspiration of mediastinal and hilar lymph nodes. Chest 2004;126(1):122–8.

16. Krasnik M, Vilmann P, Larsen SS, et al. Preliminary experience with a new method of endoscopic transbronchial real time ultrasound guided biopsy for diagnosis of mediastinal and hilar lesions. Thorax 2003;58(12):1083–6.

17. Rintoul RC, Skwarski KM, Murchison JT, et al. Endobronchial and endoscopic ultrasound-guided real-time fine-needle aspiration for mediastinal staging. Eur Respir J 2005;25(3):416–21.

18. Yasufuku K, Chiyo M, Koh E, et al. Endobronchial ultrasound guided transbronchial needle aspiration for staging of lung cancer. Lung Cancer 2005; 50(3):347–54.

19. Herth FJ, Eberhardt R, Vilmann P, et al. Real-time endobronchial ultrasound guided transbronchial needle aspiration for sampling mediastinal lymph nodes. Thorax 2006;61(9):795–8.

20. Yasufuku K, Nakajima T, Motoori K, et al. Comparison of endobronchial ultrasound, positron emission tomography, and CT for lymph node staging of lung cancer. Chest 2006;130(3):710–8.

21. Herth FJ, Ernst A, Eberhardt R. Endobronchial ultrasound-guided transbronchial needle aspiration of lymph nodes in the radiologically normal mediastinum. Eur Respir J 2006;28:910–4.

22. Shingyoji M, Nakajima T, Yoshino M, et al. Endobronchial ultrasonography for positron emission tomography and computed tomography-negative lymph node staging in non-small cell lung cancer. Ann Thorac Surg 2014;98(5):1762–7.

23. Sarwate D, Sarkar S, Krimsky WS, et al. Optimization of mediastinal staging in potential candidates for stereotactic radiosurgery of the chest. J Thorac Cardiovasc Surg 2012;144(1):81–6.

24. Liberman M, Duranceau A, Grunenwald E, et al. Initial experience with a new technique of endoscopic and ultrasonographic access for biopsy of para-aortic (station 6) mediastinal lymph nodes without traversing the aorta. J Thorac Cardiovasc Surg 2012;144(4):787–92.

25. Liberman M, Duranceau A, Grunenwald E, et al. New technique performed by using EUS access for biopsy of para-aortic (station 6) mediastinal lymph nodes without traversing the aorta (with video). Gastrointest Endosc 2011;73(5):1048–51.

26. Larsen SS, Krasnik M, Vilmann P. Endoscopic ultrasound guided biopsy of mediastinal lesions has a major impact on patient management. Thorax 2002;57:98–103.

27. Micames CG, McCrory DC, Pavey DA. Endoscopic ultrasound-guided fine-needle aspiration for non-small cell lung cancer staging: a systematic review and meta-analysis. Chest 2007;131:539–48.

28. Herth FJ, Lunn W, Eberhardt R, et al. Transbronchial versus transesophageal ultrasound-guided aspiration of enlarged mediastinal lymph nodes. Am J Respir Crit Care Med 2005;171(10):1164–7.

29. Vilmann P, Krasnik M, Larsen SS, et al. Transesophageal endoscopic ultrasound-guided fine-needle aspiration (EUS-FNA) and endobronchial ultrasound-guided transbronchial needle aspiration (EBUS-TBNA) biopsy: a combined approach in the evaluation of mediastinal lesions. Endoscopy 2005;37(9):833–9.

30. Wallace MB, Pascual JM, Raimondo M, et al. Minimally invasive endoscopic staging of suspected lung cancer. JAMA 2008;299(5):540–6.

31. Liberman M, Sampalis J, Duranceau A, et al. Endosonographic mediastinal lymph node staging of lung cancer. Chest 2014;146(2):389–97.

32. Sharples LD, Jackson C, Wheaton E, et al. Clinical effectiveness and cost-effectiveness of endobronchial and endoscopic ultrasound relative to surgical staging in potentially resectable lung cancer: results from the ASTER randomised controlled trial. Health Technol Assess 2012;16(18):1–75.

33. Szlubowski A, Zieliński M, Soja J, et al. A combined approach of endobronchial and endoscopic ultrasound-guided needle aspiration in the radiologically normal mediastinum in non-small-cell lung cancer staging — a prospective trial. Eur J Cardiothorac Surg 2010;37:1175–9.

34. Annema JT, van Meerbeeck JP, Rintoul RC, et al. Mediastinoscopy vs endosonography for mediastinal nodal staging of lung cancer: a randomized trial. JAMA 2010;304(20):2245–52.

35. Toloza EM, Harpole L, Detterbeck F, et al. Invasive staging of non-small cell lung cancer: a review of the current evidence. Chest 2003;123(1):157S–66S.

36. Von Bartheld M, van der Heijden E, Annema J. Mediastinal abscess formation after EUS-guided FNA: are patients with sarcoidosis at increased risk? Gastrointest Endosc 2012;75:1104–7.

37. Von Bartheld MB, van Breda A, Annema JT. Complication rate of endosonography (endobronchial and endoscopic ultrasound): a systematic review. Respiration 2014;87(4):343–51.

38. Liberman M, Duranceau A, Martin J, et al. Major airway laceration secondary to endobronchial ultrasound transbronchial lymph node biopsy. J Bronchology Interv Pulmonol 2010;17(3):264–5.

39. Eloubeidi MA, Tamhane A, Chen VK, et al. Endoscopic ultrasound-guided fine-needle aspiration in patients with non-small cell lung cancer and prior negative mediastinoscopy. Ann Thorac Surg 2005; 80(4):1231–9.

40. Herth FJ, Annema JT, Eberhardt R, et al. Endobronchial ultrasound with transbronchial needle aspiration for restaging the mediastinum in lung cancer. J Clin Oncol 2008;26(20):3346–50.

41. Szlubowski A, Herth FJ, Soja J. Endobronchial ultrasound-guided needle aspiration in non-small-cell lung cancer restaging verified by the transcervical bilateral extended mediastinal lymphadenectomy–a prospective study. Eur J Cardiothorac Surg 2010;37: 1180–4.

Sublobar Resection
Ongoing Controversy for Treatment for Stage I Non–Small Cell Lung Cancer

 CrossMark

Joanna Sesti, MD, Jessica S. Donington, MD, MSCR*

KEYWORDS

- Adenocarcinoma in situ • Minimally invasive adenocarcinoma • Non–small cell lung cancer
- Sublobar resection

KEY POINTS

- Improved imaging technology over the past 20 years may have rendered results of the only randomized trial on intentional sublobar resection for stage IA non–small cell lung cancer (NSCLC) outdated.
- Single-institution and population-based analyses suggest sublobar resections have equivalent outcomes to lobectomy in patients with tumors less than 2 cm and in whom adequate resection margin can be achieved.
- Data suggest sublobar resection may be a superior surgical option choice for those 75 years of age and older and those with ground glass nodules.
- Additional randomized trials exploring the intentional use of sublobar resection for stage IA NSCLC are underway, but results are many years away.

HISTORY

The optimal surgical management of early-stage non–small cell lung cancer (NSCLC) is continuously in a state of evolution. Some of the recent considerations in surgical decision making include open versus minimally invasive approaches, extent of mediastinal lymph node evaluation, use of adjuvant and neoadjuvant therapies, and extent of resection. Recent randomized trials have addressed many of these issues, but the only randomized trial comparing lobectomy to sublobar resection for stage IA NSCLC was the 1995 publication by the Lung Cancer Study Group (LCSG).[1] That trial was conducted at a time when intentional sublobar resection for good-risk patients was gaining in popularity. It was designed to prove that sublobar resections would not be inferior to lobectomies with regard to local recurrence and

cancer-free survival, but reported a 3-fold increase in local recurrence and a nonsignificant decrease in overall survival following sublobar resection. Despite the fact that a subsequent analysis decreased the significance of these differences,[2] this study standardized lobectomy as the treatment of choice for stage IA NSCLC and has guided surgical care for the past 20 years. There is a slow recognition that the findings from the landmark trial may now belong to a different era. The trial completed enrollment in 1988, before the introduction of PET with fludeoxyglucose and the widespread use of computed tomographic (CT) scans for diagnosis and staging. Improved resolution of CT scans have also allowed for detection and precise identification of subtle changes in ground glass nodules (GGNs), which paired with an improved understanding of tumor biology has

Disclosures: None.
Department of Cardiothoracic Surgery, NYU School of Medicine, 530 1st Avenue, Suite 9V, New York, NY 10016, USA
* Corresponding author.
E-mail address: jessica.donington@nyumc.org

Thorac Surg Clin 26 (2016) 251–259
http://dx.doi.org/10.1016/j.thorsurg.2016.04.007
1547-4127/16/$ – see front matter © 2016 Elsevier Inc. All rights reserved.

introduced histologic subgroups with indolent behavior and favorable outcomes. Low-dose CT scans have also served as the basis for new lung cancer screening guidelines by the US Preventive Services, which aims to detect cancers that are smaller and at an earlier stage. Simultaneously, advances in surgical technique, which allow for better tolerated resections, have brought older and poorer risk populations into consideration for anatomic resection. Each of these factors has continued to fuel the controversy over the intentional use of sublobar resection for medically fit, good-risk patients with stage IA NSCLC.

PROSPECTIVE RANDOMIZED TRIALS

There are now 2 large, multi-institutional prospective randomized trials investigating the intentional use of sublobar resections for stage IA NSCLC: one is underway in North America, Alliance/CALGB 140503,[3] and the other recently completed accrual in Japan, JCOG0802/WJOG4607,[4] but it will be many years before significant conclusions can be made from either. These trials are similar in design to the trial from the LCSG, but much larger in size and with subtle differences in inclusion and exclusion criteria (**Table 1**). The most significant difference may be the limitation in tumor size lesions less than 2 cm.

In the meantime, there is a tremendous amount of data from single-institution retrospective series and population-based analysis to help drive the controversy. Outcomes from retrospective analysis of sublobar resections can be difficult to interpret because sublobar resections are used in 2 divergent clinical settings. They can be used intentionally/electively as a parenchymal sparing option in good-risk patients with small, peripheral, or indolent tumors who would tolerate lobectomy, but they are also used as a compromise procedure in frail and debilitated patients who do not have adequate cardiopulmonary reserve to tolerate lobectomy. One of the most important questions that needs to be asked when embarking on a comparison of outcomes between lobectomy and sublobar resection for early-stage NSCLC is: "what is the specific indication for sublobar resection in this population?" Evaluating surgical outcomes in a heterogeneous population that contains both medically fit and unfit patients has limited utility because short- and long-term outcomes are significantly impacted by medical comorbidity.

POPULATION-BASED ANALYSIS

Population-based analyses are incredibly informative in situations where randomized data are lacking. They validate findings from small retrospective reviews and help define cohorts for prospective evaluations. Over the past 5 years, there have been a multitude of articles investigating the role of sublobar resection for NSCLC from the Surveillance Epidemiology and End Result (SEER) registry and the National Cancer Data Base (NCDB). SEER and NCDB are large and powerful oncologic databases, but the information collected may not be granular enough to adequately address the question of intentional sublobar resection for early-stage NSCLC because data on the indication for sublobar resection are not collected. Specifically, was a sublobar resection applied as a compromise procedure in a debilitated patient or as a parenchymal sparing option in an otherwise healthy individual? Both situations represent "curative-intent surgery," but anticipated outcomes are different. Propensity-matched analysis is frequently used to help circumvent the issue of surgical intent, but neither SEER nor the NCDB is explicit enough with regard to pulmonary disease, the primary source of comorbidity following thoracic surgery. Pulmonary function tests are not reported, and commonly used comorbidity indexes are not specific with regard to pulmonary disease. **Table 2** outlines results of recent population-based studies comparing survival between lobectomy and sublobar resections for early-stage NSCLC. At first glance, results seem contradictory, but on closer inspection, important trends become apparent. Broad comparisons of all stage I or even all stage IA patients seem to favor lobectomy over sublobar resections,[5–8] even in propensity-matched comparisons,[8] but refinements in the study populations related to older age, smaller tumor size, more indolent histology, and more recent year of treatment result in a different conclusion regarding equivalence of outcome.[5,9–12] These population-based analyses serve as important indicators that sublobar resection is likely not appropriate for all stage I NSCLC patients, but in small tumors (<2 cm), well-staged patients, and those with indolent histology, or advanced age, survival results may be equivalent.

RETROSPECTIVE ANALYSIS

Shortly after the publication from the LCSG, the University of Pittsburgh shared the results of their prospective, multicenter, nonrandomized trial of lobar versus sublobar resection. They demonstrated decreased perioperative mortality for sublobar resections, equivalent 1-year survival, and 5-year actual survival favoring lobectomy (70% vs 58%). Most deaths in this cohort were due to non–lung cancer–related causes, but they also

Table 1
Basic outline for 3 large prospective multi-institutional trials investigating intentional sublobar resection for good-risk patients with stage I non–small cell lung cancer

Trial	Years of Accrual	No.	Specific Inclusion Criteria[a]	Specific Exclusion Criteria[b]	Lobectomy Comparison	Primary Endpoint	2nd Endpoints[c]
LCSG[1]	1982–1988	276	≤3 cm, in periphery	Evidence of metastatic disease by history, physical examination, and blood chemistries; routine CT to detect occult metastases not required	Segmentectomy or wedge	DFS Local recurrence	OS Perioperative complications
JCOG0802/ WJOG4607[4]	2009–2014	1100	≤2 cm	C/T ratio <0.25 middle lobe tumors	Segmentectomy	OS	DFS Perioperative complications
Alliance/CALGB 140503[3]	2007-present	1258	≤2 cm in peripheral 1/3 of lung	Pure GGN	Segmentectomy or wedge	DFS	OS Local and systemic recurrence Prognosis by CT appearance False negative rate PET

Abbreviations: CALGB, Cancer and Lymphoma Group B; DFS, disease-free survival; JCOG, Japanese Clinical Oncology Group; OS, overall survival; WJOG, Western Japan Oncology Group.
[a] All trials have inclusion of histologically confirmed NSCLC with pathologic confirmation of N0 status, and sufficient organ function to tolerate lobectomy.
[b] All trials excluded prior malignancy and preoperative chemotherapy or radiotherapy.
[c] Postoperative pulmonary function is an endpoint of all 3 trials.

Table 2
Recent population-based analysis comparing lobectomy to sublobar resection for stage I non–small cell lung cancer

Author	Source	Population	Lobectomy Comparator	Years	Conclusion
Yendamuri et al[5]	SEER	Stage I, ≤2 cm	Segmentectomy and wedge	1988–1998	Overall survival benefit for lobectomy
Whitson et al[6]	SEER	Stage IA	Segmentectomy	1998–2007	
Shirvani et al[7]	SEER	Stage I	Sublobar resection[a]	2001–2007	
Shirvani et al[8]	SEER	Stage I	Sublobar resection[a]	2003–2009	
Speicher et al[49]	NCDB	Stage IA	Sublobar resection[a]	2003–2011	
Khuller et al[50]	NCDB	Stage IA	Sublobar resection[a]	2003–2011	
Kates et al[9]	SEER	Stage IA, ≤1 cm	Sublobar resection[a]	1988–2005	Equivalent overall survival
Yendamuri et al[5]	SEER	Stage I, ≤2 cm	Segmentectomy and wedge	1999–2004[b] 2005–2008[c]	
Wisnivesky et al[10]	SEER	Stage I ≤2 cm	Sublobar resection[a]	1998–2002	
Whitson et al[11]	SEER	AIS, MIA, or lepidic predominant ADC	Segmentectomy and wedge	1998–2007	
Razi et al[12]	SEER	Stage IA, <2 cm, age ≥75	Segmentectomy and wedge	1998–2007	

Abbreviation: ADC, adenocarcinoma.
[a] Segmentectomy and wedge resection analyzed together.
[b] Segmentectomy equivalent to lobectomy, wedge resection inferior to lobectomy.
[c] Segmentectomy and wedge equivalent to lobectomy.

documented higher rates of local/regional recurrence after sublobar resection (18% vs 4%).[13] Several other single-institution reviews echoed these results, demonstrating increased tolerability of sublobar resections, but an overall survival advantage for lobectomy. Sienel and colleagues[14] found decreased cancer-related 5-year survival and increased locoregional recurrence after segmental resection versus lobectomy

(16% and 5%, respectively) for stage IA. They attributed these findings to tumor size and width of resection. Multiple other single-institution retrospective series demonstrated comparable 5-year survival between lobectomy and sublobar resection (**Table 3**).[15–20] An interesting 3-arm analysis form Kodama and colleagues[21] compared recurrence and survival in fit patients with stage IA NSCLC undergoing "intentional" segmentectomy

Table 3
Outcomes of sublobar resection compared with lobectomy in patients with stage I non–small cell lung cancer from large retrospective analysis

Author	N	Population	Extent of Resection	5-y Survival (%)			Local Recurrence (%)			Systemic Recurrence (%)		
				SLR	Lobe	P	SLR	Lobe	P	SLR	Lobe	P
Martin-Ucar et al,[15] 2005	55	C	100% S	70	64	NS	0	12	NS	18	6	NS
El-Sherif et al,[16] 2006	784	C	41% S 59% W	40	54	.004	14	8	—	15	20	—
Kilic et al,[17] 2009	184	C	100% S	46	47	.28	6	4	.50	10	17	.28
Koike et al,[18] 2003	74	I	81% S 19% W	89	90	NS	2	1	.42	4	4	.9
Okada et al,[19] 2006	260	I	88% S 12% W	90	89	.10	5	7	NS	9	10	NS
Altorki et al,[20] 2014	327	I	30% S 70% W	86	85	.86	W: 19 S: 0	12	.15	—	—	—

Abbreviations: S, segmentectomy; W, wedge resection.

with lymph node dissection to standard lobectomy and to unfit patients undergoing "compromised" sublobar resection. Five-year survival after "intentional" limited resection was 87%, which was comparable to lobectomy at 86%. Locoregional recurrence was also comparable at 4.3%. Not surprisingly, the "intentional" sublobar group had improved overall and cancer-specific survival and locoregional control compared with the "compromised" group. These studies and others have outlined a series of prognostic tumor characteristics and resection parameters that are associated with improved rates of survival and local control after sublobar resection; these are outlined in **Table 4**.

FACTORS EFFECTING OUTCOME
Tumor Size

As far back as 1994, Warren and Faber[22] reported on a survival advantage and decreased rates of recurrence in stage I NSCLC patients with tumors less than 2 cm. Subsequent studies have noted similar results, and the 7th edition of lung cancer staging introduced the 2-cm cutoff to separate T1a and T1b tumors.[23] Subsequent analysis by Chang,[24] Mery,[25] Port,[26] and Birim[27] and their colleagues each found a significant survival improvement for stage IA tumors less than 2 cm compared with those between 2 and 3 cm.[24,28] Furthermore, survival advantage and decreased recurrence in tumors less than 2 cm treated with sublobar resection is reproducible irrespective of gender, use of invasive preoperative mediastinal staging, minimally or open surgical technique, or performance of wedge versus segmentectomy.[29–31] Several studies have shown that tumor size greater than 2 cm is an independent risk factor for recurrence in patients undergoing sublobar resection.[30–33] For this reason, the Alliance/CALGB 140503 and the JCOG0802/WJOG4607 trials each limited patient selection to tumors of 2 cm or less.[3,4]

Surgical Margin

The anatomic nature of a lobar resection does not require thoracic surgeons to typically worry about the distance from the tumor to the surgical margins, but the same is not true for sublobar resections. Although sublobar resections preserve pulmonary parenchyma and pulmonary function compared with lobectomy,[34,35] it is more difficult to determine what suffices an adequate resection margin. An R0 resection alone does not appear to be insufficient with regard to acceptable local control in NSCLC. Several studies have shown that the distance between the tumor and surgical resection margin is an important determinant of local recurrence following sublobar resection. El-Sherif and colleagues[36] analyzed the impact of distance to surgical margins in patients undergoing sublobar resection for stage I NSCLC. Tumor distances of 1 cm or larger were associated with significantly lower recurrence rates compared with margins less than 1 cm (8 vs 15%). Other groups have looked at margin:tumor ratio. A ratio of 1 or less was associated with 25% recurrence versus 6% in patients with wider margins.[37] Based on these data, The National Comprehensive Cancer Network recommends that sublobar resections achieve a resection margin of 2 cm or greater or a margin:tumor ratio 1 or greater.[38]

Segmentectomy

Sublobar resections are broken down into 2 main categories: anatomic segmentectomies and wedge resections. During segmentectomy, one or more parenchymal segments are removed with identification and division of individual segmental arteries, veins, and bronchi, and the parenchyma is divided along segmental planes. Wedge resections divide the parenchyma with no consideration of segmental anatomy and are frequently used in sublobar resections by video-assisted thoracoscopic surgery because of the relative technical ease. However, segmentectomies, although technically more challenging, facilitate more complete evaluation and removal of intralobar and hilar lymphatics, which play an important role in tumor upstaging.

Table 4 Tumor characteristics and resection specifications associated with improved survival following sublobar resection for stage I non–small cell lung cancer		
Tumor characteristics	Size	≤2 cm
	CT appearance	Pure GGN, or C/T ratio <25%
	Extent of invasion	AIS, MAI
	Location	Peripheral 1/3
Resection specifications	Extent	Segmentectomy
	Resection margin	≥1 cm, or ≥ diameter of tumor
	Mediastinal nodal evaluation	Completed

When analyzing data on survival and recurrence rates after sublobar resection, the distinction between anatomic segmentectomy and wedge resection is important. Although comparable survival rates have been shown by some groups comparing segmentectomy with lobectomy,[39] similar results have not been demonstrated for wedge resection. There is consistent evidence from retrospective series suggesting segmentectomy is associated with decreased rates of local recurrence compared with wedge resection (**Table 5**).

A series out of the Mayo Clinic by Miller and colleagues[40] looked at tumors 1 cm or smaller and rates of survival and recurrence between lobectomy, segmentectomy, and wedge resection. Although there was a survival advantage favoring lobectomy, they also noted a statistically significant survival advantage and improved local control with segmentectomy compared with wedge resection. Okada and colleagues[31] and El-Sherif and colleagues[16] each reported a critical difference in recurrence based on the extent of resection in large retrospective reviews. Sienel and colleagues[41] found significantly less local/regional recurrence (55% vs 16%) and improved cancer-specific survival (71% vs 48%) after anatomic segmentectomy with systematic nodal dissection compared with wedge resection with selective nodal sampling. It is yet to be determined whether the decreased rates of local recurrence with segmentectomy versus wedge resection are secondary to larger resection margins with segmentectomies or whether the anatomic dissection in and of itself is beneficial. The ACOSOG Z4032 trial was a multi-institutional study that evaluated the use of brachytherapy to decrease local recurrence following sublobar resection in high-risk patients. Although it reported no difference with regard to its primary endpoint, a secondary analysis noted that segmentectomy patients had larger parenchymal margins (median margin:tumor ratio was 0.76 vs 0.45), and greater number of evaluated lymph nodes and lymph node stations than those who underwent wedge. The more complete nodal evaluation also resulted in an increased rate of nodal upstaging of 9% versus 1% between segmentectomy and wedge resection groups.[33]

SPECIAL CONSIDERATIONS
The Elderly Patient

The elderly patient presents a particularly interesting population in the discussion of sublobar resection for early-stage NSCLC. Advanced age appears to reduce the importance of local control and increase importance of tolerability and preserved pulmonary function. Retrospective series from Kilic and colleagues[17] and Dell'Amore and colleagues[42] independently demonstrated decreased perioperative morbidity and equivalent overall survival in patients 75 years of age and older who underwent sublobar resection as compared with lobectomy. A recent analysis of the SEER database limited to patients aged 75 or older with stage IA NSCLC showed no significant difference in 5-year cancer-specific survival for patients with T1a tumors between wedge, segmentectomy (hazard ratio [HR]: 1.009), or lobar resections (HR: 0.98).[12]

Table 5
Outcomes of wedge resection versus anatomic segmentectomy in stage I non–small cell lung cancer

Author, Year	N	Extent of Resection	MLND (%)	Local Recurrence Rate (%)		5-y Cancer-specific Survival (%)	
				W	S	W	S
Miller et al,[40] 2002	100	12 S 13 W	94	30	8	42	75
Okada et al,[31] 2005	1272	285 S 64 W	100	N/R	N/R	97 (<2 cm) 39 (2–3 cm) 0 (>3 cm)	92 (<2 cm) 85 (2–3 cm) 63 (>3 cm)
El-Sherif et al,[16] 2006	81	26 S 55 W	74	15	4	N/R	N/R
Sienel et al,[41] 2008	87	56 S 31 W	100 S Selective W	55	16	48	71

Abbreviations: MLND, mediastinal lymph node evaluation; N, number; N/R, not reported; S, segmentectomy; W, wedge resection.

Ground Glass Nodules

The understanding of biologic heterogeneity of lung adenocarcinomas has evolved dramatically in the past 20 years since the LCSG publication. These are no longer viewed as a group of homogeneous group tumors whose prognosis is predicted primarily by size and nodal involvement, but rather a heterogeneous group with indolent and aggressive subtypes with pathologic and radiologic correlates. This evolution began with increased resolution of cross-sectional imaging, which allowed for visualization of part-solid and GGN. The histologic classification of pulmonary adenocarcinoma by the International Association for the Study of Lung Cancer, American Thoracic Society, and European Respiratory Society[43] further organized this biologic heterogeneity. Adenocarcinoma in situ (AIS) and minimally invasive adenocarcinoma (MIA) describe small (<3 cm), solitary adenocarcinomas consisting of purely lipidic growth without invasion or less than 0.5-cm invasion. These adenocarcinomas represent a distinct group with absence of nodal involvement and 100% disease-specific survival following resection. The ability to recognize and describe these lesions with low malignant potential is shifting what is considered curable treatment. Where once lobectomy with systematic mediastinal lymph node evaluation was the standard for all, there is a growing mindset that parenchymal-sparing options may be a superior treatment alternative, especially because these tumors have a greater predilection for the development of additional GGNs than nodal or systemic spread, which increases the importance of pulmonary parenchyma preservation. An essential factor that allows for use of an intentional sublobar resection for these minimally invasive tumors is the ability to accurately identify them preoperatively. Retrospective series suggest radiographic markers such as tumor disappearance ratio greater than 50%[44] or greater than 75%,[45] or consolidation to tumor size (C/T) ratio less than 0.25[46] can be predictive. A prospective evaluation from Japan (JCOG0201) was designed to accurately identify patients for intentional sublobar resection.[47] It found tumors 2 cm or less with a C/T ratio less than or equal to 0.25 was highly predictive of diagnosis of noninvasive adenocarcinoma. Reports from specialized centers have also suggested that intraoperative frozen section can be used to rule out the presence of an invasive adenocarcinoma when treating a GGN.[48] When AIS, MAI, and adenomatous hyperplasia are grouped together, the diagnostic accuracy of frozen section was impressive, with less than 0.5% of prospectively evaluated patients undergoing an "inadequate" resection due to underestimation of invasive components on frozen section. Although one can question the reproducibility of these findings outside of highly specialized facilities, frozen section could serve as an important adjunct in the decision to perform a resection less than lobectomy or defer mediastinal lymph node evaluation in an otherwise healthy individual.

SUMMARY

Optimal treatment of early-stage NSCLC has come a long way since the original LCSG trial that established lobectomy as the treatment of choice for the past 20 years. The use of sublobar resection for early-stage NSCLC continues to be a point of considerable debate. Although the results of the Alliance/CALGB 140503 and the JCOG0802/WJOG4607 trials are still awaited, there are various well-designed single-institution studies that have reinforced the value of sublobar resection for early-stage NSCLC. Evidence suggests that sublobar resections should be considered in well-selected patients with small (<2 cm), peripheral tumors, and in whom an adequate resection margin (>2 cm or margin:tumor >1) can be guaranteed, and that they may be a superior choice for those 75 years and older and with pure GGNs. In general, segmentectomy seems to afford better oncologic results than simple wedge resection and should be prioritized based on the expertise of the surgeon.

REFERENCES

1. Ginsberg RJ, Rubinstein LV. Randomized trial of lobectomy versus limited resection for T1 N0 non-small cell lung cancer. Lung Cancer Study Group. Ann Thorac Surg 1995;60:615–22 [discussion: 622–3].
2. Lederle FA. Lobectomy versus limited resection in T1 N0 lung cancer. Ann Thorac Surg 1996;62: 1249–50.
3. Available at: https://clinicaltrials.gov/ct2/show/record/NCT00499330. Accessed May 02, 2016.
4. Nakamura K, Saji H, Nakajima R, et al. A phase III randomized trial of lobectomy versus limited resection for small-sized peripheral non-small cell lung cancer (JCOG0802/WJOG4607L). Jpn J Clin Oncol 2010;40:271–4.
5. Yendamuri S, Sharma R, Demmy M, et al. Temporal trends in outcomes following sublobar and lobar resections for small (</=2 cm) non-small cell lung cancers—a Surveillance Epidemiology End Results database analysis. J Surg Res 2012;183(1):27–32.
6. Whitson BA, Groth SS, Andrade RS, et al. Survival after lobectomy versus segmentectomy for stage I

non-small cell lung cancer: a population-based analysis. Ann Thorac Surg 2011;92:1943–50.

7. Shirvani SM, Jiang J, Chang JY, et al. Comparative effectiveness of 5 treatment strategies for early-stage non-small cell lung cancer in the elderly. Int J Radiat Oncol Biol Phys 2012;84:1060–70.

8. Shirvani SM, Jiang J, Chang JY, et al. Lobectomy, sublobar resection, and stereotactic ablative radiotherapy for early-stage non-small cell lung cancers in the elderly. JAMA Surg 2014;149(12):1244–53.

9. Kates M, Swanson S, Wisnivesky JP. Survival following lobectomy and limited resection for the treatment of stage I non-small cell lung cancer <= 1 cm in size: a review of SEER data. Chest 2011;139:491–6.

10. Wisnivesky JP, Henschke CI, Swanson S, et al. Limited resection for the treatment of patients with stage IA lung cancer. Ann Surg 2010;251:550–4.

11. Whitson BA, Groth SS, Andrade RS, et al. Invasive adenocarcinoma with bronchoalveolar features: a population-based evaluation of the extent of resection in bronchoalveolar cell carcinoma. J Thorac Cardiovasc Surg 2012;143:591–600.e1.

12. Razi SS, John MM, Sainathan S, et al. Sublobar resection is equivalent to lobectomy for T1a non-small cell lung cancer in the elderly: a Surveillance, Epidemiology, and End Results database analysis. J Surg Res 2016;200:683–9.

13. Landreneau RJ, Sugarbaker DJ, Mack MJ, et al. Wedge resection versus lobectomy for stage I (T1 N0 M0) non-small-cell lung cancer. J Thorac Cardiovasc Surg 1997;113:691–8 [discussion: 698–700].

14. Sienel W, Stremmel C, Kirschbaum A, et al. Frequency of local recurrence following segmentectomy of stage IA non-small cell lung cancer is influenced by segment localisation and width of resection margins–implications for patient selection for segmentectomy. Eur J Cardiothorac Surg 2007;31:522–7 [discussion: 527–8].

15. Martin-Ucar AE, Nakas A, Pilling JE, et al. A case-matched study of anatomical segmentectomy versus lobectomy for stage I lung cancer in high-risk patients. Eur J Cardiothorac Surg 2005;27:675–9.

16. El-Sherif A, Gooding WE, Santos R, et al. Outcomes of sublobar resection versus lobectomy for stage I non-small cell lung cancer: a 13-year analysis. Ann Thorac Surg 2006;82:408–15 [discussion: 415–6].

17. Kilic A, Schuchert MJ, Pettiford BL, et al. Anatomic segmentectomy for stage I non-small cell lung cancer in the elderly. Ann Thorac Surg 2009;87:1662–6 [discussion: 1667–8].

18. Koike T, Yamato Y, Yoshiya K, et al. Intentional limited pulmonary resection for peripheral T1 N0 M0 small-sized lung cancer. J Thorac Cardiovasc Surg 2003;125:924–8.

19. Okada M, Koike T, Higashiyama M, et al. Radical sublobar resection for small-sized non-small cell lung cancer: a multicenter study. J Thorac Cardiovasc Surg 2006;132:769–75.

20. Altorki NK, Yip R, Hanaoka T, et al. Sublobar resection is equivalent to lobectomy for clinical stage 1A lung cancer in solid nodules. J Thorac Cardiovasc Surg 2014;147:754–62 [discussion: 762–4].

21. Kodama K, Doi O, Higashiyama M, et al. Intentional limited resection for selected patients with T1 N0 M0 non-small-cell lung cancer: a single-institution study. J Thorac Cardiovasc Surg 1997;114:347–53.

22. Warren WH, Faber LP. Segmentectomy versus lobectomy in patients with stage I pulmonary carcinoma. Five-year survival and patterns of intrathoracic recurrence. J Thorac Cardiovasc Surg 1994;107:1087–93 [discussion: 1093–4].

23. Rami-Porta R, Ball D, Crowley J, et al. The IASLC Lung Cancer Staging Project: proposals for the revision of the T descriptors in the forthcoming (seventh) edition of the TNM classification for lung cancer. J Thorac Oncol 2007;2:593–602.

24. Chang MY, Mentzer SJ, Colson YL, et al. Factors predicting poor survival after resection of stage IA non-small cell lung cancer. J Thorac Cardiovasc Surg 2007;134:850–6.

25. Mery CM, Pappas AN, Burt BM, et al. Diameter of non-small cell lung cancer correlates with long-term survival: implications for T stage. Chest 2005;128:3255–60.

26. Port JL, Kent MS, Korst RJ, et al. Tumor size predicts survival within stage IA non-small cell lung cancer. Chest 2003;124:1828–33.

27. Birim O, Kappetein AP, Takkenberg JJ, et al. Survival after pathological stage IA nonsmall cell lung cancer: tumor size matters. Ann Thorac Surg 2005;79:1137–41.

28. Mery CM, Pappas AN, Bueno R, et al. Similar long-term survival of elderly patients with non-small cell lung cancer treated with lobectomy or wedge resection within the surveillance, epidemiology, and end results database. Chest 2005;128:237–45.

29. Bando T, Miyahara R, Sakai H, et al. A follow-up report on a new method of segmental resection for small-sized early lung cancer. Lung Cancer 2009;63:58–62.

30. Fernando HC, Santos RS, Benfield JR, et al. Lobar and sublobar resection with and without brachytherapy for small stage IA non-small cell lung cancer. J Thorac Cardiovasc Surg 2005;129:261–7.

31. Okada M, Nishio W, Sakamoto T, et al. Effect of tumor size on prognosis in patients with non-small cell lung cancer: the role of segmentectomy as a type of lesser resection. J Thorac Cardiovasc Surg 2005;129:87–93.

32. Bando T, Yamagihara K, Ohtake Y, et al. A new method of segmental resection for primary lung

cancer: intermediate results. Eur J Cardiothorac Surg 2002;21:894–9 [discussion: 900].

33. Kent M, Landreneau R, Mandrekar S, et al. Segmentectomy versus wedge resection for non-small cell lung cancer in high-risk operable patients. Ann Thorac Surg 2013;96(5):1747–54 [discussion: 1754–5].

34. Keenan RJ, Landreneau RJ, Maley RH Jr, et al. Segmental resection spares pulmonary function in patients with stage I lung cancer. Ann Thorac Surg 2004;78:228–33 [discussion: 233].

35. Harada H, Okada M, Sakamoto T, et al. Functional advantage after radical segmentectomy versus lobectomy for lung cancer. Ann Thorac Surg 2005; 80:2041–5.

36. El-Sherif A, Fernando HC, Santos R, et al. Margin and local recurrence after sublobar resection of non-small cell lung cancer. Ann Surg Oncol 2007; 14:2400–5.

37. Schuchert MJ, Pettiford BL, Keeley S, et al. Anatomic segmentectomy in the treatment of stage I non-small cell lung cancer. Ann Thorac Surg 2007;84:926–32 [discussion: 932–3].

38. Ettinger DS, Akerley W, Borghaei H, et al. Non-small cell lung cancer, version 2.2013. J Natl Compr Canc Netw 2013;11:645–53 [quiz: 653].

39. Yoshikawa K, Tsubota N, Kodama K, et al. Prospective study of extended segmentectomy for small lung tumors: the final report. Ann Thorac Surg 2002;73:1055–8 [discussion: 108–9].

40. Miller DL, Rowland CM, Deschamps C, et al. Surgical treatment of non-small cell lung cancer 1 cm or less in diameter. Ann Thorac Surg 2002;73: 1545–50 [discussion: 1550–1].

41. Sienel W, Dango S, Kirschbaum A, et al. Sublobar resections in stage IA non-small cell lung cancer: segmentectomies result in significantly better cancer-related survival than wedge resections. Eur J Cardiothorac Surg 2008;33:728–34.

42. Dell'Amore A, Monteverde M, Martucci N, et al. Early and long-term results of pulmonary resection for non-small-cell lung cancer in patients over 75 years of age: a multi-institutional study. Interact Cardiovasc Thorac Surg 2013;16:250–6.

43. Travis WD, Brambilla E, Noguchi M, et al. International Association for the Study of Lung Cancer/American Thoracic Society/European Respiratory Society International Multidisciplinary Classification of Lung Adenocarcinoma. J Thorac Oncol 2011;6: 244–85.

44. Shimada Y, Yoshida J, Hishida T, et al. Predictive factors of pathologically proven noninvasive tumor characteristics in T1aN0M0 peripheral non-small cell lung cancer. Chest 2012;141:1003–9.

45. Takahashi M, Shigematsu Y, Ohta M, et al. Tumor invasiveness as defined by the newly proposed IASLC/ATS/ERS classification has prognostic significance for pathologic stage IA lung adenocarcinoma and can be predicted by radiologic parameters. J Thorac Cardiovasc Surg 2014;147:54–9.

46. Nitadori J, Bograd AJ, Morales EA, et al. Preoperative consolidation-to-tumor ratio and SUVmax stratify the risk of recurrence in patients undergoing limited resection for lung adenocarcinoma ≤2 cm. Ann Surg Oncol 2013;20:4282–8.

47. Suzuki K, Koike T, Asakawa T, et al. A prospective radiological study of thin-section computed tomography to predict pathological noninvasiveness in peripheral clinical IA lung cancer (Japan Clinical Oncology Group 0201). J Thorac Oncol 2011;6: 751–6.

48. Liu S, Zhang Y, Li Y, et al. Precise diagnosis of intraoperative frozen section is an effective method to guide resection strategy for peripheral small-sized lung adenocarcinoma. J Clin Oncol 2015;34(4): 307–13.

49. Speicher PJ, Gu L, Gulack BC, et al. Sublobar resection for clinical stage IA non-small-cell lung cancer in the United States. Clin Lung Cancer 2016;17(1):47–55.

50. Khullar OV, Liu Y, Gillespie T, et al. Survival after sublobar resection versus lobectomy for clinical stage ia lung cancer: an analysis from the National Cancer Data Base. J Thorac Oncol 2015;10:1625–33.

Stereotactic Body Radiation Therapy for Stage I Non–Small Cell Lung Cancer

 CrossMark

Paul Aridgides, MD*, Jeffrey Bogart, MD

KEYWORDS

- Stereotactic body radiation therapy • SBRT • Stage I non–small cell lung cancer • NSCLC
- Medically inoperable • Medically operable

KEY POINTS

- Stereotactic body radiation therapy (SBRT) for stage I non–small cell lung cancer is well-tolerated with excellent local control.
- Prospective trials in medically inoperable patients support improved survival with SBRT compared with historical cohorts with conventional fractionated radiotherapy.
- Although encouraging data continue to emerge for SBRT in medically operable patients, the inherent limitations in these analyses (patient selection, large database studies) must be considered when interpreting these results, given the difficulty in completing a randomized phase III comparison with surgical resection.
- Although SBRT toxicity is generally mild, for central tumors there is a risk of severe complications and the optimal fractionation scheme for safe and effective SBRT delivery is the subject of ongoing investigation.
- Several dosimetric guidelines have been established to lower the risk of skin and rib toxicity for peripheral tumors.

INTRODUCTION

Stereotactic body radiation therapy (SBRT) typically involves delivery of high doses of radiation per fraction (10–20 Gy) in a few (3–5) fractions to a small target (<5 cm). This technique relies on technological advances in image-guided radiation therapy to visualize the tumor both before and during treatment delivery, as well as account for respiratory motion. Early-stage non–small cell lung carcinoma (NSCLC) has proven to be a well-suited disease population for the development of this technique,[1] as immobilization with abdominal compression was used to minimize respiratory motion, and daily visualization of a placed fiducial allowed radiographic verification of the target. Additionally, patients with medically inoperable stage I NSCLC experienced mixed outcomes following conventional radiotherapy with curative intent.[2] The encouraging local control and manageable toxicity observed in medically inoperable patients has led to widespread adoption of SBRT in the United States[3] as well as globally, where it is also referred to as stereotactic ablative radiotherapy.[4] The aim of this article was to discuss the development of SBRT as a technology for inoperable and operable patients with stage 1 NSCLC. Treatment characteristics,

Disclosures: None.
Department of Radiation Oncology, SUNY Upstate Medical University, 750 E Adams Street, Syracuse, NY 13210, USA
* Corresponding author.
E-mail address: aridgidp@upstate.edu

Thorac Surg Clin 26 (2016) 261–269
http://dx.doi.org/10.1016/j.thorsurg.2016.04.008
1547-4127/16/$ – see front matter © 2016 Elsevier Inc. All rights reserved.

thoracic.theclinics.com

including dose and tumor location, and how they pertain to local control and toxicity, respectively, are reviewed in the context of published and ongoing research.

MEDICALLY INOPERABLE PATIENTS
Development of Stereotactic Body Radiation Therapy Technique

Timmerman and colleagues[1] published the results of a phase I SBRT dose escalation trial at the University of Indiana in 2003. Thirty-seven medically inoperable patients with stage I NSCLC received 3 fractions starting with 800 cGy × 3, with increases of 200 cGy per fraction for each subsequent cohort until the maximum tolerated dose (MTD) was established. The definition of medically inoperable used was for tumors that were technically resectable; however, patients were poor candidates for surgery based on pulmonary function testing and/or blood gas measurements. Treatment was delivered with computed tomography (CT)-based planning, immobilization with a rigid stereotactic body frame, abdominal compression to minimize respiratory motion, and placement of a fiducial marker before treatment that was imaged daily for target verification. As such, expansions for treatment planning were limited to 1.0 cm from gross tumor volume (GTV) to planning tumor volume (PTV) in the superior-inferior direction and 0.5 cm radially.

Using a tumor size cutoff (≤ 7 cm) and stratification (T1 vs T2), investigators reported that with 6000 cGy at 2000 cGy per fraction, an MTD was not reached. With continued dose escalation, an MTD of 66 Gy was established for T2 (>3 cm) tumors; however, T1 (≤ 3 cm) tumors were not treated above 60 Gy.[5] In T2 patients with tumors ≥ 5 cm who received 72 Gy, 3 of 5 patients experienced grade 3 to 4 toxicity (pneumonitis in 2 patients and tracheal necrosis in 1 patient). Treatment was otherwise well-tolerated and local control was encouraging, particularly for doses ≥ 54 Gy where only 1 local failure was observed. Subsequent institutional retrospective series of SBRT for medically inoperable stage I NSCLC were likewise favorable with 80% to 95% local control.[6,7] Given the risk of severe and potentially fatal toxicity seen with SBRT for central tumors,[8] the Radiation Therapy Oncology Group (RTOG) excluded tumors within 2 cm of the proximal bronchial tree for study under the 3-fraction (54 Gy total) regimen.

Prospective Collaborative Trials

A multi-institutional phase II trial from the Scandinavian countries of Sweden, Denmark, and Norway evaluated SBRT in 57 patients with medically inoperable stage I NSCLC.[9] Criteria for inoperability included chronic obstructive pulmonary disease by published criteria (65%) or cardiovascular disease (35%). Pathologic confirmation of malignancy was not required, with 33% of patients diagnosed clinically by imaging characteristics. The SBRT regimen consistent of 45 Gy in 15-Gy fractions prescribed to the 67% isodose line.

The Scandinavian prospective trial demonstrated a 3-year local control rate of 92% following SBRT. Regional relapses were observed in 5% of patients and distant relapse in 16%. Although most patients had T1 (70%) as opposed to T2 (30%) tumors, all cases of progression were in T2 patients. T2 disease was estimated to have a 41% risk of combined failure (local, regional, or distant), in comparison with 18% for T1 tumors ($P = .027$). Treatment was well-tolerated with 16 patients (28%) experiencing grade 3 toxicity, and no reported grade 5 events.

In a seminal phase II trial, RTOG 0236, 55 patients with medically inoperable stage I NSCLC were treated with SBRT to 60 Gy in 3 fractions.[10] Detailed quality assurance included central review of treatment planning for the first patient enrolled at a participating center. Enrollment required evaluation by a thoracic surgeon or pulmonologist to determine a patient medically inoperable. Criteria used included pulmonary function testing, blood gas measurements, and presence of severe medical comorbidities.

The outcomes following SBRT in RTOG 0236 were favorable, with 3-year tumor control of 98% for the primary site and 3-year locoregional control of 87%. Disseminated metastases developed in 11 patients (22%). The median survival was 48 months, with rare cases of severe toxicity (4% grade 4) and no fatal events. Long-term results of RTOG 0236 were recently reported showing a 5-year primary tumor failure rate of 7% and 5-year overall survival of 40%.[11] There was a 20% rate of recurrence in the primary site or involved lobe at 5 years. Although there were only 11 patients with T2 tumors in the study cohort, the metastasis rate for T2 tumors was 47%.[10] Although this merits further investigation, this is consistent with inferior outcomes for T2 patients on the Scandinavian trial.[9]

Prospective trials reporting long-term outcomes for SBRT in stage I NSCLC are summarized in **Table 1**. The favorable results and toxicity profile seen in RTOG 0236 support the use of protocol guidelines for SBRT delivery.[11] Tumor margins included 1 cm in the superior-inferior directions and 0.5 cm radially to define a PTV. Timing considerations include 40 hours between treatments and completion within 14 days.

Table 1
Results of stereotactic body radiation therapy for stage I non–small cell lung cancer in selected prospective trials with long-term (3-year) outcomes

	Patient Population	Treatment Regimen	Local Control 3-y/5-y	Overall Survival 3-y/5-y
RTOG 0236[10,11] Prospective phase 2	55 patients 100% inoperable T1 80%, T2 20% 100% biopsy proven	54 Gy, 3 fractions Prescribed for 95% coverage PTV	98%/93% (primary tumor) 91%/80% (involved lobe)	56%/40%
Scandinavian[9] Prospective phase 2	57 patients 100% inoperable T1 70%, T2 30% 67% biopsy proven	45 Gy in 3 fractions Prescribed to tumor periphery	92%/NA	60%/NA
JCOG 0403[14] Prospective phase 2	164 patients 61% inoperable, 39% operable T1 100% 100% biopsy proven	48 Gy in 4 fractions Prescribed to isocenter	87%/NA (inoperable) 85%/NA (operable)	60%/NA (inoperable) 77%/NA (operable)

Abbreviations: JCOG, Japanese cooperative oncology group; NA, not available for 5 year results; PTV, planning tumor volume; RTOG, radiation therapy oncology group.

Treatment planning required 95% coverage of the PTV with prescription dose. It should be noted that for planning with lung heterogeneity corrections, the prescription dose was more accurately calculated to be 54 Gy.

MEDICALLY OPERABLE PATIENTS
Retrospective Experience

SBRT programs were largely developed to improve the efficacy of medically inoperable patients and as such treatment was generally targeted toward that patient population. Nevertheless, even early on in the development of the technique, select patients who otherwise would qualify as being eligible for standard surgical resection with lobectomy were treated with SBRT as they apparently had refused surgery. Although it is difficult to define the specific reason that operable patients were treated with SBRT in retrospective series, patients choosing SBRT may be more likely to be older and have comorbidities compared with surgical cohorts. Many patients also may decide to have SBRT for a second primary lung cancer if they have had surgical resection in the past.

Several retrospective studies have reported favorable outcomes with sublobar resection (SLR) or SBRT in select patients who were otherwise candidates for lobectomy. One of the largest retrospective experiences comes from a Japanese multi-institutional database including a total of 87 patients, median age 74, who were medically operable but refused surgery.[12] A range of SBRT fractionation regimens was used and the total

dose was 45.0 to 72.5 Gy given in 3 to 10 fractions with a median calculated biological effective dose of 116 Gy. Patients were treated between 1995 and 2004, such that the median follow-up was reasonably long at the time of analysis. Overall 5-year local control rates for T1 and T2 tumors were 92% and 73%, respectively, and 5-year overall survival rates were 72% and 62%, respectively. There was only a single grade 3 toxicity, keeping in mind it is often difficult to assess toxicity and causality in a retrospective analysis. The investigators concluded that SBRT appeared safe in the operable population with overall survival appearing similar to surgical series.

A report from a large single institutional database from VU University in the Netherlands included 177 patients, 60% T1 and 40% T2, deemed to be medically operable.[13] This represented approximately 25% of all patients treated with SBRT. Similar to the Japanese experience, the median age of 76 years was older than would be typical for surgical series. A total dose of 60 Gy was used and the number of fractions given was dependent on tumor location. The median follow-up was shorter than the Japanese series at 31.5 months, although intermediate-term outcomes were excellent with 3-year overall survival and local tumor control of 84.7% and 93.0%. Regional and distant failure rates at 3 years were each 9.7%. Grade 3 radiation pneumonitis and rib fractures were in 2% and 3%, respectively. Although most patients treated did not have a histologic diagnosis, the 3-year survival rate of 96% was excellent for the subset of 59 patients with a histologic diagnosis.

Prospective Phase II Trials

Modest-size prospective phase II trials of SBRT for standard-risk patients have been completed in Japan and the United States. Data from these studies are just now maturing, but long-term results may provide for a more "accurate" rate of local tumor control given that median survival (and median follow-up) would be expected to be longer in the standard risk population.

Mature outcomes from the Japan Cooperative Oncology Group (JCOG) phase II 0403 trial were recently published.[14] The trial included 64 operable patients treated with SBRT to a dose of 48 Gy in fractions prescribed to the isocenter. The study tended to enroll elderly patients and the median age overall was 79 years. After a median follow-up of 67 months, 3-year absolute local tumor control was 85.4% and 3-year overall survival was 76.5%. Progression-free survival, local progression-free survival, and event-free survival at 3 years were 68.6%, 54.5%, and 51.4%, respectively. Treatment was fairly well tolerated with 5 patients experiencing severe (grade 3) toxicity, including 2 patients with radiation pneumonitis. Interestingly, regional lymph node failures were noted in 16 patients, although only 4 patients had isolated nodal relapse. A comparison to the Japanese Lung Cancer Registry suggested similar overall survival at 3 and 5 years compared with surgically treated stage I disease, particularly when the analysis was restricted to patients 80 years and older.[14,15] The initial results of the prospective RTOG 0618 trial, which was restricted to those deemed as operable after assessment by a thoracic surgeon, have been presented. The SBRT dose was 54 Gy in 3 fractions prescribed to an appropriate isodose line covering the planning target volume. The median age of 72 years was younger than the JCOG 0403 trial. After a median follow-up of 25 months, the estimated 2-year primary tumor failure rate for 26 eligible patients was 7.7%.[16] The 2-year estimates of progression-free survival and overall survival were 65.4% and 84.4%, respectively. Treatment was again reasonably well tolerated with 4 patients experiencing grade 3 adverse events and without grade 4 or 5 toxicity. These series provide an initial sense of the utility of SBRT for operable patients; the data generated may help guide future prospective studies. For example, the JCOG experience suggests more intensive SBRT regimens might be considered for operable patients (compared with the Japanese standard 48 Gy in 4 fractions) and also call into question whether more intensive nodal staging should be routinely considered for operable patients.

Randomized Phase III Trials

Attempts to compare surgical resection and SBRT in a randomized setting have been challenging, and although phase III trials have been initiated for both medically operable and medically inoperable patients, none have been completed. Nevertheless, a recent combined analysis of 2 phase III studies, the STARS and ROSEL trials, which compared SBRT and lobectomy for operable stage I disease, was published.[17] Between the 2 trials, 58 patients were enrolled and randomly assigned to either SBRT (n = 31) or to surgery (n = 27). After median follow-up ranging from 35 to 40 months, 6 patients in the surgery group died, including 2 from cancer progression and 1 related to surgery, as compared with 1 death in those randomized to SBRT. Estimated 3-year overall survival and recurrence-free survival with SBRT were 95% and 86% compared with 79% and 80% in the surgery group. The difference in overall survival significantly favored SBRT in the STARS trial but not in ROSEL. There were 4 patients with regional nodal recurrence in the SBRT group compared with a single nodal recurrence in the surgery group, likely reflecting the requirement for lymph node sampling or dissection in the surgical group. Although the results of this combined analysis are provocative, the overall impact is limited, given the small number of patients accrued to each trial.

Large Database Analyses

Given the difficulty in completing randomized trials to address the question of surgical treatment versus SBRT, several large analyses have recently been published in an attempt to shed light on the question. Although the findings are often interesting and thought provoking, all are subject to inherent limitations of the databases studied, including the potential for significant bias in patient selection. Many series are further complicated by inclusion of both medically operable and medically inoperable patients. Multiple reviews of Surveillance, Epidemiology, and End Results have been performed. Interpretations have varied with demonstration of similar outcomes regardless of treatment when propensity matching is performed,[18] whereas other analyses suggesting long-term results might be superior with surgery particularly when segmental resection is used.[19] The largest database analysis to date included more than 100,000 patients treated between 1998 and 2010 in the National Cancer Data Base (NCDB). Median overall survival favored the surgery group, but only 5% of patients in the analysis were treated with SBRT and the relative contribution of patient selection or better cancer control could not be determined given the limitations of NCDB.[20] This analysis is again limited by the time frame encompassed, as very few patients actually received SBRT during the early part of the study. In the end, the relative efficacy of surgery and SBRT can be determined only with a prospective clinical trial, which unfortunately has been challenging to complete.

TOXICITY CONSIDERATIONS WITH STEREOTACTIC BODY RADIATION THERAPY
Skin and Chest Wall/Rib

Investigators at Memorial Sloan Kettering Cancer Center evaluated the risk of skin toxicity in a prospectively database of 50 patients treated from 2006 to 2008.[21] Although grade 1 toxicity was common (38%), grade 2 toxicity was observed in 8% of patients and severe toxicity was rare but possible (grade 3 in 4%, grade 4 in 2%). Factors associated with grade ≥ 2 toxicity included tumor distance from posterior chest wall <5 cm and skin dose $\geq 50\%$ prescription. Reflective of the early era of SBRT in this analysis was the observation that treatment limited to 3 beams was also associated with increased risk of toxicity; SBRT plans with 3 beams are not likely to be used in contemporary treatment. However, in the RTOG 0236 trial, which established a reasonable standard for SBRT technique, skin toxicity grades 1 to 3 was still apparent in 13% of patients.[10]

In a pooled retrospective analysis from the University of Virginia and the University of Colorado, parameters for the development of chest wall pain or rib fracture were studied in 60 patients with peripheral tumors.[22] Inclusion required a tumor within 2.5 cm from the chest wall and/or a chest wall dose of greater than 20 Gy. Grade 3 chest wall pain was observed in 17 patients (28%) and rib fracture in 5 patients (8%). The chest wall volume receiving 30 Gy (V30) best predicted the risk of severe toxicity with a recommendation to limit the chest wall V30 to less than 30 mL.

In a retrospective analysis of 134 patients who all received SBRT with 60 Gy in 3 fractions, Stephans and colleagues[23] found a correlation between late (≥ 6 weeks post SBRT) chest wall toxicity and the volume of chest wall receiving 30 to 60 Gy (V30 to V60). Examples of chest wall toxicity included chest pain, as well as skin reaction; however, asymptomatic rib fractures were excluded. Late toxicity was mild and limited to 10 patients (4 grade 1 and 6 grade 2). The investigators suggested chest wall treatment parameters of V30 ≤ 30 mL and V60 ≤ 3 mL.

Representative treatment plans from 2 patients with peripheral lesions receiving 48 Gy in 4 fractions, using either 3-dimensional conformal radiation (3DCRT) (**Fig. 1**) or intensity-modulated radiation therapy (IMRT) (**Fig. 2**), are shown. For patient 1, who was treated in 2011 with 3DCRT, the primary tumor imaging was consistent with evolving radiation changes; however, a subsequent fracture developed in the nearby rib that was treated conservatively. IMRT may be able to decrease the rib or chest wall dose for peripheral lesions compared with 3DCRT.

Central Location

Special caution is required with the use of SBRT for central tumors due to risk of severe toxicity. In a phase II trial from the Indiana University of 70 patients, SBRT was a possible contributing factor in 6 patient deaths.[8] Four of these deaths were also receiving treatment for bacterial pneumonia. Apparent deaths from central SBRT included complications from a pericardial effusion in a tumor adjacent to the superior mediastinum, and massive hemoptysis following SBRT for a carinal tumor in a patient who also had local recurrence. Perihilar or central tumor location was a predictor of grade 3 to 5 toxicity on multivariate analysis ($P = .004$) and associated with a 2-year freedom from severe toxicity of only 54%.

For the RTOG 0236 trial of SBRT to 60 Gy in 3 fractions, tumors within 2 cm of proximal bronchial tree were excluded. Perhaps as a result, there were only 7 cases (13%) of grade 3 toxicity and 2 cases (4%) of grade 5 toxicity.[10] There were no deaths attributed to SBRT. As an alternative to 3 fractions of 18 to 20 Gy for central tumors, RTOG 0813 has studied the safety of 5-fraction SBRT in a phase I/II dose escalation trial. The initial dose of 10 Gy × 5 fractions was subsequently increased in 0.5 Gy/fraction increments, as long as safety endpoints were met, with successful dose escalation to 60 Gy in 12-Gy fractions. In the first reports of toxicity in abstract form, death due to hemoptysis occurred in 4% of patients at a mean of 13 months post SBRT (range 5.5–14 months). (Bezjak World Lung abstract 2015).[24]

The optimal treatment of central tumors, including which patients are candidates for SBRT and in what fractionation, is yet to be determined. Further analysis of the RTOG 0813 trial is awaited, in which grade 5 hemoptysis was seen at multiple dose levels (10.5, 11.5, and 12 Gy). In contrast, there were no deaths reported after SBRT in 4 fractions (40–50 Gy) in 13 patients with central and superior tumors in an M.D. Anderson Cancer Center analysis.[25] Given that both prospective and retrospective cases of treatment death following a 5-fraction SBRT regimen have been

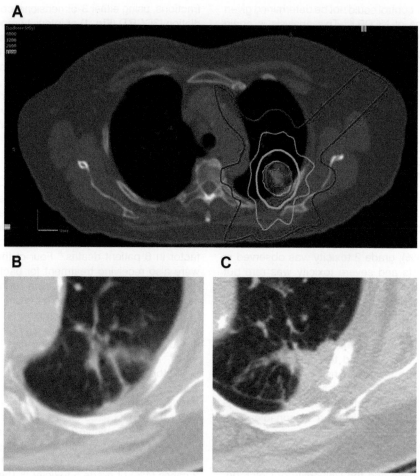

Fig. 1. SBRT plan with 3DCRT (*A*). Targets are GTV in red and PTV in cyan. Representative isodose lines in centigray are magenta (4800 cGy), green (3200 cGy), orange (2000 cGy), and blue (1000 cGy). Rib volume receiving 3200 cGy is 4 mL. The RTOG 0915 rib constraint is that less than 1 mL receives 3200 cGy, although this may be exceeded for cases in which the PTV lies within the rib volume (as with this patient). Surveillance CT imaging reveals evolving radiation changes in the lung parenchyma at 1 year (*B*) and 3 years (*C*) post SBRT. At 3 years, there are sclerotic changes and possible rib fracture.

reported,[26] caution is advised before adoption to standard practice.

Pulmonary Toxicity

Even in a patient population with significant medical comorbidities and poor pulmonary function, pulmonary toxicity following SBRT is generally mild. In the RTOG 0236 trial, although grade 1 to 2 pulmonary adverse events occurred in 24 (44%) patients, moderate or severe toxicity was uncommon (15% grade 3, and 2% grade 4).[10] Grade 1 to 2 events were not protocol specified for prospective evaluation, and due to mild nature, difficult to quantify. In an updated analysis of pulmonary toxicity on RTOG 0236, pneumonitis occurred in 16% of patients and all cases were grade 1 to 3.[27] SBRT was not found to be

associated with clinically significant changes in pulmonary function testing (PFT), even for patients with poor baseline lung function. A decreased diffusion capacity following SBRT, which had been observed previously,[28] was not associated with corresponding changes in blood oxygenation. Poor lung function should not be used to preclude SBRT treatment, and this subset actually demonstrated improved overall survival in comparison with patients who had normal PFTs but were inoperable for cardiac comorbidity.

OPTIMAL STEREOTACTIC BODY RADIATION THERAPY DOSE

Although the optimal dose/fractionation is the subject of ongoing investigation, evidence exists to support a relationship between dose and tumor

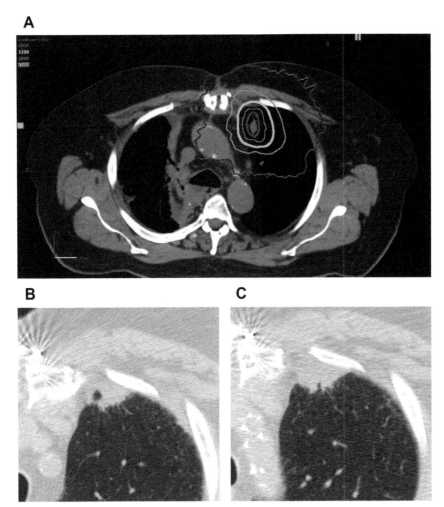

Fig. 2. SBRT plan with IMRT (*A*). Targets are GTV in red and PTV in cyan. Representative isodose lines in centigray are magenta (4800 cGy), green (3200 cGy), orange (2000 cGy), and blue (1000 cGy). Rib dose is improved with use of IMRT compared with 3DCRT (see **Fig. 1**). Rib dose receiving 3200 cGy (green) is 0.6 mL (RTOG 0915 constraint, <1 mL receives 3200 cGy). Surveillance CT imaging at 1 year (*B*) and 1.5 years (*C*) shows evolving radiation changes in lung parenchyma without evidence of rib injury, although longer follow-up is still required.

control.[29] In the phase I dose escalation study at the University of Indiana, there was only 1 local failure observed in patients receiving ≥54 Gy as compared with 9 local failures at doses of 24 to 48 Gy.[5] In a large multicenter retrospective study of 257 patients, investigators from Japan demonstrated improved local control and overall survival with SBRT regimens of a biologically effective dose (BED) ≥100 Gy.[30] The most common regimen of 48 Gy in 4 fractions had a calculated BED of 106 Gy. For the 60 Gy/3 fraction regimen, the BED was calculated to be 180 Gy. In a retrospective analysis from the Cleveland Clinic, there was no difference in tumor control between 50 Gy/5-fraction (BED = 100 Gy) or 60 Gy/3-fraction regimens.[31]

Evidence suggests the feasibility of single-fraction SBRT to doses of 30 to 34 Gy.[32] In a phase 1 dose escalation trial from Stanford, the single-fraction SBRT dose was successfully increased from 15 Gy to 30 Gy.[33] There was an apparent improvement in local control with 25 or 30 Gy compared with lower doses. Increased toxicity was more common with central tumors and in the setting of prior thoracic radiation, with the investigators advising against high-dose single-fraction SBRT in these patients. In the NRG Oncology RTOG 0915 phase 2 trial, medically inoperable patients with peripheral stage I NSCLC were randomized to SBRT with either 34 Gy in 1 fraction or 48 Gy in 4 fractions.[34] The primary endpoint was the rate of grade 3 or higher adverse events at 1 year. Although both arms met the pre-specified criteria of both 1 year local control greater than 90% and the 1-year rate of grade ≥ 3 adverse events $\leq 17\%$, according to the trial design the 34 Gy in 1 fraction was the superior regimen based on a numerically lower adverse event rate (10.3% vs 13.3%). The 1-year primary tumor control was 97% for 34 Gy and 91% for 48 Gy. Overall survival and disease-free survival at 2 years were higher with 48 Gy (78% overall survival and 71% disease-free survival) compared with 34 Gy (61% overall survival and 56% disease-free survival); however, confidence intervals were overlapping. Although continued follow-up is warranted with regard to the nonsignificant trend of survival difference, the investigators recommended a phase 3 comparison of 34 Gy in 1 fraction to the 3-fraction regimen (54–60 Gy) of RTOG 0236, with the primary endpoint of overall survival.

SUMMARY

SBRT is an acceptable standard of care for medically inoperable stage I NSCLC. Randomized trials comparing surgery with SBRT for medically operable patients have unfortunately failed to accrue. Multidisciplinary evaluation is helpful to tailor personalized therapeutic recommendations of lobectomy, SLR, or SBRT for appropriate patients with stage I NSCLC. For patients who are medically operable but refuse surgery, emerging prospective data for the use of SBRT are encouraging, although trials have been limited in size. The optimal dose and fractionation for SBRT is the subject of ongoing investigation. A modification of SBRT scheme is recommended for central tumors, where severe toxicity (albeit rare) has been reported even following more conservative regimens.

REFERENCES

1. Timmerman R, Papiez L, McGarry R, et al. Extracranial stereotactic radioablation: results of a phase I study in medically inoperable stage I non-small cell lung cancer. Chest 2003;124(5): 1946–55.
2. Sibley GS, Jamieson TA, Marks LB, et al. Radiotherapy alone for medically inoperable stage I non-small-cell lung cancer: the Duke experience. Int J Radiat Oncol Biol Phys 1998;40(1):149–54.
3. Pan H, Simpson DR, Mell LK, et al. A survey of stereotactic body radiotherapy use in the United States. Cancer 2011;117(19):4566–72.
4. Lo SS, Slotman BJ, Lock M, et al. The development of stereotactic body radiotherapy in the past

decade: a global perspective. Future Oncol 2015; 11(19):2721–33.
5. McGarry RC, Papiez L, Williams M, et al. Stereotactic body radiation therapy of early-stage non-small-cell lung carcinoma: phase I study. Int J Radiat Oncol Biol Phys 2005;63(4):1010–5.
6. Nyman J, Johansson KA, Hulten U. Stereotactic hypofractionated radiotherapy for stage I non-small cell lung cancer–mature results for medically inoperable patients. Lung Cancer 2006;51(1):97–103.
7. Videtic GM, Stephans K, Reddy C, et al. Intensity-modulated radiotherapy-based stereotactic body radiotherapy for medically inoperable early-stage lung cancer: excellent local control. Int J Radiat Oncol Biol Phys 2010;77(2):344–9.
8. Timmerman R, McGarry R, Yiannoutsos C, et al. Excessive toxicity when treating central tumors in a phase II study of stereotactic body radiation therapy for medically inoperable early-stage lung cancer. J Clin Oncol 2006;24(30):4833–9.
9. Baumann P, Nyman J, Hoyer M, et al. Outcome in a prospective phase II trial of medically inoperable stage I non-small-cell lung cancer patients treated with stereotactic body radiotherapy. J Clin Oncol 2009;27(20):3290–6.
10. Timmerman R, Paulus R, Galvin J, et al. Stereotactic body radiation therapy for inoperable early stage lung cancer. JAMA 2010;303(11):1070–6.
11. Timmerman RD, Hu C, Michalski J, et al. Long-term results of RTOG 0236: a phase II trial of stereotactic body radiation therapy (SBRT) in the treatment of patients with medically inoperable stage I non-small cell lung cancer. Int J Radiat Oncol Biol Phys 2014;90(1):S30.
12. Onishi H, Shirato H, Nagata Y, et al. Stereotactic body radiotherapy (SBRT) for operable stage I non-small-cell lung cancer: can SBRT be comparable to surgery? Int J Radiat Oncol Biol Phys 2011; 81(5):1352–8.
13. Lagerwaard FJ, Verstegen NE, Haasbeek CJ, et al. Outcomes of stereotactic ablative radiotherapy in patients with potentially operable stage I non-small cell lung cancer. Int J Radiat Oncol Biol Phys 2012;83(1):348–53.
14. Nagata Y, Hiraoka M, Shibata T, et al. Prospective trial of stereotactic body radiation therapy for both operable and inoperable T1N0M0 non-small cell lung cancer: Japan clinical oncology group study JCOG0403. Int J Radiat Oncol Biol Phys 2015; 93(5):989–96.
15. Asamura H, Goya T, Koshiishi Y, et al. A Japanese lung cancer registry study: prognosis of 13,010 resected lung cancers. J Thorac Oncol 2008;3(1):46–52.
16. Timmerman RD, Harvey RP, Pass I, et al. RTOG 0618: Stereotactic body radiation therapy (SBRT) to treat operable early-stage lung cancer patients. J Clin Oncol 2013;31(Suppl):2013 [abstract: 7523].

17. Chang JY, Senan S, Paul MA, et al. Stereotactic ablative radiotherapy versus lobectomy for operable stage I non-small-cell lung cancer: a pooled analysis of two randomised trials. Lancet Oncol 2015;16(6): 630–7.

18. Shirvani SM, Jiang J, Chang JY, et al. Lobectomy, sublobar resection, and stereotactic ablative radiotherapy for early-stage non-small cell lung cancers in the elderly. JAMA Surg 2014;149(12):1244–53.

19. Ezer N, Veluswamy RR, Mhango G, et al. Outcomes after stereotactic body radiotherapy versus limited resection in older patients with early-stage lung cancer. J Thorac Oncol 2015;10(8):1201–6.

20. Puri V, Crabtree TD, Bell JM, et al. Treatment outcomes in stage I lung cancer: a comparison of surgery and stereotactic body radiation therapy (SBRT). J Thorac Oncol 2015;10(12):1776–84.

21. Hoppe BS, Laser B, Kowalski AV, et al. Acute skin toxicity following stereotactic body radiation therapy for stage I non-small-cell lung cancer: who's at risk? Int J Radiat Oncol Biol Phys 2008;72(5):1283–6.

22. Dunlap NE, Cai J, Biedermann GB, et al. Chest wall volume receiving >30 Gy predicts risk of severe pain and/or rib fracture after lung stereotactic body radiotherapy. Int J Radiat Oncol Biol Phys 2010;76(3): 796–801.

23. Stephans KL, Djemil T, Tendulkar RD, et al. Prediction of chest wall toxicity from lung stereotactic body radiotherapy (SBRT). Int J Radiat Oncol Biol Phys 2012;82(2):974–80.

24. Bezjak A, Paulus R, Gaspar L. NRG Oncology/RTOG 0813 Trial of Stereotactic Body Radiotherapy (SBRT) for Central Tumors – Adverse Events. Journal of Thoracic Oncology 2015;10(9):S210.

25. Chang JY, Balter PA, Dong L, et al. Stereotactic body radiation therapy in centrally and superiorly located stage I or isolated recurrent non-small-cell lung cancer. Int J Radiat Oncol Biol Phys 2008; 72(4):967–71.

26. Corradetti MN, Haas AR, Rengan R. Central-airway necrosis after stereotactic body-radiation therapy. N Engl J Med 2012;366(24):2327–9.

27. Stanic S, Paulus R, Timmerman RD, et al. No clinically significant changes in pulmonary function following stereotactic body radiation therapy for early-stage peripheral non-small cell lung cancer: an analysis of RTOG 0236. Int J Radiat Oncol Biol Phys 2014;88(5):1092–9.

28. Henderson M, McGarry R, Yiannoutsos C, et al. Baseline pulmonary function as a predictor for survival and decline in pulmonary function over time in patients undergoing stereotactic body radiotherapy for the treatment of stage I non-small-cell lung cancer. Int J Radiat Oncol Biol Phys 2008; 72(2):404–9.

29. Roach MC, Videtic GM, Bradley JD, et al. Treatment of peripheral non-small cell lung carcinoma with stereotactic body radiation therapy. J Thorac Oncol 2015;10(9):1261–7.

30. Onishi H, Shirato H, Nagata Y, et al. Hypofractionated stereotactic radiotherapy (HypoFXSRT) for stage I non-small cell lung cancer: updated results of 257 patients in a Japanese multi-institutional study. J Thorac Oncol 2007;2(7 Suppl 3):S94–100.

31. Stephans KL, Djemil T, Reddy CA, et al. A comparison of two stereotactic body radiation fractionation schedules for medically inoperable stage I non-small cell lung cancer: the Cleveland Clinic experience. J Thorac Oncol 2009;4(8):976–82.

32. Videtic GM, Stephans KL, Woody NM, et al. 30 Gy or 34 Gy? Comparing 2 single-fraction SBRT dose schedules for stage I medically inoperable non-small cell lung cancer. Int J Radiat Oncol Biol Phys 2014;90(1):203–8.

33. Le QT, Loo BW, Ho A, et al. Results of a phase I dose-escalation study using single-fraction stereotactic radiotherapy for lung tumors. J Thorac Oncol 2006;1(8):802–9.

34. Videtic GM, Hu C, Singh AK, et al. A randomized phase 2 study comparing 2 stereotactic body radiation therapy schedules for medically inoperable patients with stage I peripheral non-small cell lung cancer: NRG oncology RTOG 0915 (NCCTG N0927). Int J Radiat Oncol Biol Phys 2015;93(4): 757–64.

Management of Stage IIIA (N2) Non–Small Cell Lung Cancer

Erin A. Gillaspie, MD, Dennis A. Wigle, MD, PhD*

KEYWORDS

- Stage IIIA • Non–small cell lung cancer • PORT • Adjuvant • Neoadjuvant • Surgery • N2

KEY POINTS

- There is no consensus as to the optimal management of IIIA (N2) non–small cell lung cancer, nor for the role of surgery in treating this disease stage.
- Clinical trial evidence struggles to keep up with technology advancement and the evolution of expert opinion.
- Despite advances in chemotherapeutic regimens, methods of delivery for radiation, and less invasive surgical techniques, survival for patients with stage IIIA (N2) malignancies remains poor.
- Further developments in both will stimulate and maintain controversy in the field for years to come.

BACKGROUND

Approximately 15% of patients with non–small cell lung cancer (NSCLC) will present with stage IIIA (N2) disease.[1] The optimal management of patients with stage IIIA (N2) NSCLC disease remains widely debated among surgeons, pulmonologists, and oncologists. Many trials have set out to determine the optimal combination and timing of multimodality treatment. Such trials have historically been challenged by accrual issues and relevance to modern practice by the time of publication. Unfortunately, this leaves many aspects of patient care for IIIA (N2) disease unclear.

Despite advances in chemotherapeutic regimens, methods of delivery for radiation, and less invasive surgical techniques, survival for patients with stage IIIA (N2) malignancies remains poor. Here, the current literature evaluating neoadjuvant and adjuvant therapies, surgical indications, and new immunomodulators in the context of their relevance to the treatment of IIIA (N2) disease is reviewed.

STAGING CONSIDERATIONS

Stage IIIA (N2) NSCLC is a varied mix of tumor sizes and nodal involvement. Tumors vary dramatically from subcentimeter to being greater than 7 cm or invading surrounding structures such as the chest wall. Nodal involvement, although defined as N2 or ipsilateral mediastinal, also varies significantly. Survival outcome and treatment considerations for single-station, microscopic disease are very different from multistation, bulky nodal disease (**Table 1**).

Accurate Determination of IIIA (N2) Non–Small Cell Lung Cancer

Appropriate staging of lung cancer is essential, because treatment recommendations and prognosis vary significantly by stage. Even with a thorough preoperative workup, there will still be a percentage of patients who will have occult mediastinal disease at the time of surgery that will become clear only on final pathology.

Division of Thoracic Surgery, Mayo Clinic, 200 First Street, Rochester, MN 55905, USA
* Corresponding author.
E-mail address: wigle.dennis@mayo.edu

Thorac Surg Clin 26 (2016) 271–285
http://dx.doi.org/10.1016/j.thorsurg.2016.04.001
1547-4127/16/$ – see front matter

Table 1			
Seventh edition lung cancer staging: stage IIIA			
Stage IIIA	T1a	N2	M0
	T1b	N2	M0
	T2a	N2	M0
	T2b	N2	M0
	T3	N1	M0
	T3	N2	M0
	T4	N0	M0
	T4	N1	M0

Initial Staging

Computed tomography (CT) scanning, a standard part of the workup for lung cancer, is the least sensitive and specific modality for the identification of lymph node involvement. The utility of PET scanning has evolved and now holds an important role for extrathoracic staging in ruling out distant metastasis, which would render a patient unresectable. However, confirmation of PET scan abnormalities with tissue diagnosis remains important because the study also carries a significant rate of false positive upstaging.[2]

Endobronchial ultrasound (EBUS) with transbronchial needle aspiration has increasingly been used as a favored method for diagnosis of suspicious mediastinal nodes. Review of available publications reveals a median sensitivity of 89%, although values range in the literature from 46% to 97%.[2]

Mediastinoscopy was considered the gold-standard diagnostic technique for the assessment of mediastinal lymph nodes for decades. Although replaced in many centers by EBUS as the first line for mediastinal assessment, mediastinoscopy remains an important tool, with a sensitivity of 89% and specificity of 100%.[2]

How Do Endobronchial Ultrasound and Mediastinoscopy Compare?

Yasafuku and colleagues[3] presented their findings at the American Association for Thoracic Surgery in 2011. The study enrolled 153 patients who underwent EBUS followed directly by mediastinoscopy, with an average of 3 to 4 nodal stations sampled by EBUS per patient. They found no significant difference between EBUS-TBNA and mediastinoscopy in determining the pathologic N stage. There were no complications from EBUS-TBNA, while mediastinoscopy had minor complications in 2.6% of patients. They concluded EBUS-TBNA could safely replace mediastinoscopy for mediastinal staging in potentially resectable patients.

How transferable these results are to routine practice remains unknown. Procedural proficiency is certainly a confounding factor for both EBUS and mediastinoscopy, and it will be important to confirm these and other results in a broader setting. Furthermore, it will be important to sort out where endoscopic staging works best and which cases best benefit from mediastinoscopy, such as the dilemma of how best to restage a patient after receiving neoadjuvant therapy.[4]

Unfortunately, even guidelines for mediastinal assessment are debated, with some physicians favoring routine sampling of all lymph node stations, whereas others favor sampling of only those nodes that are suspicious on imaging. Thorough sampling is most important in central tumors with radiographically normal-appearing nodes. When nodes are grossly abnormal, these can be sampled initially and are much more likely to yield a positive diagnosis, in some cases obviating sampling additional areas.[5] The authors remain committed at their institution to an approach of routine sampling of all lymph node stations to accomplish thorough preoperative staging.

Occult N2 Disease

Even with negative imaging, negative surgical biopsy, and a small (T1) cancer, there will still be a subset of patients found to have occult N2 disease on frozen section at the time of lung resection or discovered later on final pathology.

The rate of occult N2 disease with T1 primary tumors and negative imaging is in the range of 4% to 6%, and 9% to 10% for T2 tumors. In clinical stage I patients, higher risk features for N2 disease include central tumors, larger T size, and positive N1 disease.[6,7] Prediction models to try to determine the risk of N2 disease have been developed and tested, although are not widely accepted and adopted.[8,9]

Is Restaging Necessary After Neoadjuvant Therapy?

"Restaging" has different definitions depending on the investigator's perspective and the medical or surgical subspecialty involved. To some, restaging represents an imaging-based evaluation to rule out distant metastases that would render surgery a futile exercise for improving survival. For many, this involves a more comprehensive workup, including pathologic reassessment of the mediastinum to determine if there is persistent disease, given the known improvement in survival for resected patients, wherein mediastinal sterilization has been achieved.

Veeramachaneni and colleagues[10] surveyed thoracic surgeons in practice in an anonymous Web-based surgery to determine practice patterns related to single station N2 disease. Twenty percent of surgeons in the study responded that they would proceed with resection of single-station disease after neoadjuvant therapy regardless of mediastinal nodal response.

Repeat mediastinoscopy, particularly in the setting of radiation therapy, can be challenging. Most studies evaluating the safety of repeat mediastinoscopy found that it could be accomplished safely and with high yield in experienced hands. However, when compared with first-time mediastinoscopy, it does carry an increased morbidity and mortality (1% vs 0.05%).[11] A further dilemma is the challenge of accurate diagnosis of residual cancer in the context of significant treatment effect. This setting is a potentially important setting in which to further study the efficacy and use of EBUS versus mediastinoscopy.

With improved imaging technology, studies have emerged attempting to correlate a specific standardized uptake value (SUV) with the likelihood of finding persistent cancer within diseased lymph nodes. Although some have focused on absolute value of SUV, others have examined the change in SUVmax as the best predictor of pathologic response. Although a potentially useful measure, studies to date have suggested relatively poor sensitivity and specificity overall for residual PET activity to correctly identify persistent tumor.[12]

There is unfortunately no consensus as to what studies should be included in restaging, and what degree of residual disease should be considered for resection. The approach in many centers typically comes down to what is considered "resectable" or "unresectable" disease, with imaging and other diagnostic tests directed toward accurate determination of this status for an individual patient.

Who Can Tolerate a Multimodality Treatment Regimen?

In many cases, patients with lung cancer are older, long-time smokers with compromised lung function. They may be frail and deconditioned from the cancer itself or other comorbid medical conditions. Surgery, chemotherapy, and radiotherapy each have risks associated with the therapy that can be cumulative in the multimodality setting, and careful multidisciplinary review of each patient is important to determine the best individualized treatment regimen.

An important factor to consider in all patients presenting with lung cancer is their overall fitness to be able to tolerate any proposed treatment regimen.

Surgery certainly carries well-known morbidity and mortality. However, there are also nontrivial complications related to chemotherapy and radiation that are underappreciated, particularly in the cumulative context of a multimodality treatment regimen. Although many symptoms and consequences of treatment are reversible, they can result in interruptions or prolongation of therapy, which is associated with decreased survival.[13] The most common morbidities include neutropenia, esophagitis, pneumonitis, respiratory complications, and significant nausea or emesis.[14] The reported rate of treatment associated mortality of chemotherapy or radiation therapy alone for locally advanced NSCLC is 2%. Concurrent therapy mortality ranges in the literature from 2.3% to 4.9%.[14,15]

There is a paucity of literature stratifying comorbid conditions and risks of treatments for patients with lung cancer. With more complex and aggressive regimens, careful consideration should be given to each patient to determine the ability to complete the outlined treatment regimen determined best suited for the individual patient.

THE EVOLUTION OF MULTIMODALITY TREATMENT FOR LOCALLY ADVANCED LUNG CANCER

Neoadjuvant therapy as part of a multimodality treatment of lung cancer has been in evolution since the 1980s. Two highly influential studies, Rosell and colleagues[16] published in the *New England Journal of Medicine* in 1994 and Roth and colleagues[17] published in the *Journal of the National Cancer Institute* also in 1994, prominently influenced the landscape of neoadjuvant treatment for stage IIIA (N2) disease.

Rosell and colleagues[16] studied 60 patients with stage IIIA (N2) NSCLC randomized to receive surgery alone versus chemotherapy followed by surgery. A median survival of 26 months was achieved in patients undergoing multimodality treatment versus 8 months in the surgery-alone group. Disease-free survival was also improved in the patients who received chemotherapy. Roth and colleagues[17] from MD Anderson Cancer Center also studied 60 patients and found that after neoadjuvant chemotherapy, a significant rate of major clinical response was achieved in 35%, and the median survival was 64 months for chemotherapy plus surgery versus 11 months for surgery alone.

Both studies closed early because of the marked improvement in survival seen in patients undergoing neoadjuvant chemotherapy.

The Southwest Oncology Group (SWOG),[18] the French Thoracic Cooperative Group,[19] and the European Organization for Research and Treatment of Cancer[20] all sponsored similar trials, which confirmed the benefits of neoadjuvant chemotherapy in disease-free survival and overall survival when comparing chemotherapy plus surgery to surgery alone.

The use of neoadjuvant chemotherapy and the concept of a multimodality treatment approach for known N2 disease have subsequently become a standard therapeutic approach. Many phase II and III clinical trials have since emerged to try to determine which combination of agents and treatment schedule provides the greatest benefit.

The concept of concurrent chemoradiation being better than sequential treatment was forwarded by publication of several papers studying the concept for unresectable locally advanced NSCLC disease in the late 1990s.[21,22] Despite increased toxicity, extrapolation of these data to multimodality regimens involving surgery began to be considered as a means to enhance treatment effect.

Radiation Dosage in the Neoadjuvant Setting

In 1993, The Fox Chase Cancer Center[23] published results of a phase II study to determine the feasibility and safety of pulmonary resection after concurrent chemotherapy and radiation. Patients received a platinum-based chemotherapy regimen and concurrent high-dose radiation to 60 Gy. Results from 13 patients were presented with a postoperative complication rate of 62% (8/13), which included 3 bronchopleural fistulas and a mortality of 23% (3/13). Given these findings, the investigators raised concerns regarding the safety of their treatment regimen, suspecting that radiation-induced pulmonary toxicity accounted for the unacceptably high rate of respiratory complications perioperatively. The results of this study would be quoted for many years and discouraged the use of definitive dose radiation (60 Gy) in patients who might potentially go on to surgery.

Phase II Trials of Neoadjuvant Concurrent Chemoradiation

The role of neoadjuvant chemotherapy with concurrent radiation therapy to 45 Gy followed by surgical resection in stage IIIA (N2) NSCLC was initially studied in the SWOG 8805 trial.[24] Importantly, the trial was able to demonstrate that trimodality therapy was feasible, toxicity was acceptable, and survival was double what was expected in patients undergoing radiation therapy alone. They also reported that the best predictor

of overall survival for patients was a pathologically negative mediastinum on final pathology.

Intergroup 0139–Definitive or Just Old News?

The Intergroup 0139 trial[25] was a prospective phase III trial that sought to determine the utility of surgical resection after concurrent chemoradiation for stage IIIA lung cancer.

The study randomized patients with T1-3 N2 disease to receive either induction chemotherapy plus 45 Gy radiation followed by surgery if no progression or uninterrupted radiation to a total of 61 Gy. Approximately 200 patients were randomized to each treatment arm.

Although the study did not demonstrate a statistically significant difference in survival for the patients receiving trimodality therapy involving surgery, there were several interesting findings in subset analysis. Patients with N0 status at the time of resection had an improved overall survival compared with those who had residual mediastinal nodal disease. Pneumonectomy carried a concerningly high mortality (26%) and overall worse outcomes compared with patients undergoing lobectomy. Disease-free survival was however higher in the trimodality arm.

In a controversial subgroup analysis, patients with tumors that were resectable with lobectomy following chemoradiation to 45 Gy had improved survival compared with patients undergoing chemoradiation alone. Interestingly, the overall survival curves cross with late separation at 5 years, indicating a trend toward improved overall survival with trimodality therapy, although this did not reach statistical significance. The initial lower survival in the trimodality arm is largely attributable to excess mortality in the initial postoperative period related to patients undergoing pneumonectomy.

On final pathology, it was also found that chemoradiation to 45 Gy had a measurable complete response rate in those patients who went on to have resection (14% of patients were T0N0).

A summary of key findings of the article are as follows:

- Patients with N0 status at the time of thoracotomy following induction treatment had an improved overall 5-year survival than those who have residual mediastinal nodal disease.
- Patients undergoing pneumonectomy following induction chemoradiation to 45 Gy had worse treatment-related and overall outcomes when compared with patients undergoing lobectomy.
- Chemoradiation to 60 Gy (without surgery) had a measurable cure rate.

- Chemotherapy and concurrent radiotherapy with and without resection are both acceptable treatment options for N2 NSCLC with measurable cure rates.
- Patients with tumors that are resectable with lobectomy following chemoradiation (to 45 Gy) may have improved outcomes when compared with patients undergoing chemoradiation alone (to 60 Gy).

The results of the INT 0139 trial remain controversial, with disparate interpretations from surgeons, medical oncologists, and radiation oncologists as to the value of trimodality therapy and the respective role for treating disciplines involved.

EVOLUTION OF TREATMENT IN THE MODERN ERA: INTERGROUP 0139 AFTERMATH
The Role of Surgery

The role of surgery in the management of N2 disease remains controversial to this day.

Physicians who favor definitive chemotherapy and radiation argue that no study has definitely proven a survival benefit for adding surgery to multimodality treatment regimens for N2 disease. When taken at face value, the INT 0139 trial specifies no statistically significant difference in survival with the addition of surgery. Although exceedingly high pneumonectomy mortality was certainly a confounding factor to these results, this has not swayed detractors.

Who Should be Considered for Surgery: Not All N2 Is Created Equally

Patient survival in stage IIIA (N2) is dictated not only by the presence of mediastinal nodes but also by the extent of nodal involvement. A French study by Andre and colleagues[26] published in 2000 reviewed the survival of 702 patients from 6 centers. They found that N2 disease treated by surgery alone had a 5-year survival of 34% for microscopic, single-station, 11% for macroscopic, single-station, and only 3% for macroscopic, multistation disease.

Although few stage IIIA patients are currently treated with single-modality therapy in the modern era, this study highlights several very important facts. There is significant variability in patients presenting with N2 disease, and patient selection for surgery remains an essential part of decision making and should be made part of a multidisciplinary team. Stratification of predicted survival for N2 patients must impact surgical treatment decisions, with patients achieving mediastinal sterilization having the best outcomes, and those with bulky, multistation disease having the worst independent of the treatment regimen applied. What this information unfortunately does not provide is a clear cutoff for who may benefit from a surgical approach, often leaving other factors to sway decision making in an individualized manner based on how treating physicians interpret the available clinical trial data. Although patients achieving mediastinal sterilization have the best overall outcomes, patients with residual N2 disease are theoretically in a position to benefit from adding surgical resection as further local therapy to a chemoradiation regimen leaving persistent residual disease. The 5-year survival for this subgroup having residual nodal disease at the time of surgery after chemoradiation involving 45 Gy was approximately 25% in the INT 0139 study.

Is Surgery Safe After Neoadjuvant Chemoradiation to 60 Gy?

Despite the initial biases that developed as a consequence of the small Fox Chase study and the safe use of 45 Gy in clinical trial treatment arms, many studies have gone on to show that operating after 60 Gy of radiation can be done safely.

The Radiation Therapy Oncology Group (RTOG) 0229 combined neoadjuvant carboplatin and paclitaxel with concurrent radiotherapy to a total dose of 61.2 Gy, followed by surgical resection. Fifty-six patients enrolled in the trial; 43 had mediastinal nodal restaging and 37 went on to have surgical resection. The rate of complete pathologic response in mediastinal nodes was 63% compared with the 50% found in the SWOG 8805 trial. Further confirming the benefits of mediastinal clearance, the study reported a 2-year survival of 75% versus 52% in patients with persistent nodal involvement. Importantly, they also demonstrated no increased surgical morbidity or mortality related to the higher dose of radiation.[27]

Outcomes of surgery after 45 Gy and 60 Gy were studied at the Mayo Clinic. Patients with stage IIIA (N2) disease were studied retrospectively. All received trimodality therapy. The study found that high-dose induction radiation was not associated with increased risk of postoperative morbidity, mortality, or hospital length of stay. Surgery was shown to be safely performed following any level of radiation therapy.[28]

University of Alabama similarly found no increased incidence of morbidity or mortality operating after 60 Gy of radiation. They highlighted the additional benefit of providing uninterrupted maximum medical therapy for all patients regardless of whether they are ultimately selected to undergo resection.[29]

These prospective and other retrospective studies suggest there may be more differences in patient-specific responses and individualized radiation treatment plans in the context of surgical resection than in the overall difference in morbidity between 45 Gy and 60 Gy as a total radiation dose. One emerging treatment strategy from these observations is the use of chemoradiation to 60 Gy for all patients, deferring decisions about surgical resection until after restaging 4 to 6 weeks following completion of treatment. This practice prevents breaks in therapy after 45 Gy, allows all patients to receive an acceptable treatment regimen even if surgery is not pursued, and facilitates the careful selection of patients deemed most likely to benefit from surgery in multidisciplinary review, despite this remaining undefined and unstudied.

Outcomes of Surgery for Stage IIIA (N2)

Single-center and multicenter trials have emerged confirming both the safety and the potential survival benefits of surgery for patients with N2 disease.

The European Organisation for Research and Treatment of Cancer [30] in a phase III randomized, multicenter trial studied the outcomes of 579 patients with pathologically proven N2 disease. All patients received neoadjuvant chemotherapy, and responders to the chemotherapy were then randomized to receive radiation therapy or surgery ± radiation therapy. Overall 5-year survival in the surgery group was 15.7% versus 14% in the radiation group and did not reach statistical significance.

Cerfolio and colleagues[31] studied 402 patients within their institution who presented with non-bulky N2 disease, all diagnosed preoperatively. Despite the obvious selection bias, several interesting observations are noted. Eighty-one percent of patients were able to complete their neoadjuvant treatments. Approximately 49% of patients ultimately returned for restaging, and 57% of those went on for resection. On multivariate analysis, patients younger than 70, extent of lymph node involvement, and response to neoadjuvant therapy dictated who ultimately went to the operating room for R0 resection. Overall 5-year survival of the cohort was 13.2%; however, overall 5-year survival ranged from 4.8% in patients who did not complete neoadjuvant chemotherapy to 53% in patients who had complete pathologic response of their nodes. The outcome for patients with residual N2 disease (partial response) approaching that of complete responders is particularly interesting (**Table 2**).

Table 2 Survival with surgery as part of multimodality therapy	
Treatment	**5-y Survival (%)**
Incomplete neoadjuvant therapy	4.8
Chemoradiation alone	17
Neoadjuvant therapy and surgery with unsuspected recalcitrant N2	42
Neoadjuvant therapy and surgery with partial response	49
Neoadjuvant therapy and surgery with complete response	53

Data from Cerfolio RJ, Maniscalco L, Bryant AS. The treatment of patients with stage IIIA non-small cell lung cancer from N2 disease: who returns to the surgical arena and who survives. Ann Thorac Surg 2008;86(3):912–20.

Darling and colleagues[32] retrospectively reviewed 215 patients with stage IIIA (N2) disease who were treated with neoadjuvant chemoradiation (cisplatin/etoposide and 45 Gy) followed by surgery or definitive chemoradiation (cisplatin/etoposide and 61 Gy). Surgical patients had a median survival of 4.2 years versus 1.7 years. There were 6 deaths in the surgery group, 5 of whom had undergone pneumonectomy. Recurrence occurred in 54.8% of surgical patients versus 73.9% of nonsurgical patients. They concluded that in an appropriate patient population, surgery enhances both disease-free and overall survival. They caution, however, that not all N2 disease is equivalent. Patients with bulky mediastinal disease were excluded from this study, and all their patients had an excellent performance status (majority Eastern Cooperative Oncology Group 0 or 1).

Specific Surgical Considerations

Persistent N2 disease

Complete pathologic response and nodal downstaging after neoadjuvant therapy have been shown to provide patients with the best long-term survival in patients who undergo surgical resection.

However, not all patients will have complete response; some will have partial response, and some will have stable disease with no progression. These patients may still derive some benefit when their treatment regimen includes surgery compared with chemotherapy and radiation alone, with some studies showing increased time to recurrence and improved overall.[26]

The question remains, however, how much residual disease after neoadjuvant therapy is too much disease to obtain benefit from surgical resection. Should microscopic single-station only be considered, or macroscopic single-station, or microscopic multistation? Furthermore, focused studies will be required to determine which patient subsets with N2 disease truly benefit from the addition of surgery to their overall treatment regimen.

Incidentally discovered N2

The availability and accuracy of mediastinal imaging continue to improve. Unfortunately, no preoperative study is 100% sensitive and specific in identifying N2 disease. Performing mediastinoscopy on all patients, in particular for clinical stage I, has been shown to have a low yield and lacks cost-effectiveness, and a survival advantage has not been demonstrated.[33] There is also an incidence of patients who will have a negative mediastinoscopy, video-assisted thoracoscopic surgery, or open lymph node sampling and go on to have one or more positive N2 nodes on final pathology.[34]

When confronted with unforeseen N2 disease at the time of thoracotomy or thoracoscopy with potentially resectable disease IIIA (N2) disease, many surgeons will complete resection of the tumor if feasible and refer their patient for consideration of adjuvant therapy, given the patient has already been subjected to the morbidity of general anesthesia and chest incisions. This approach can be reasonable given the known benefit of adjuvant chemotherapy and a re-emerging role for PORT in IIIA (N2) disease.

Is a pneumonectomy really too dangerous to be considered after radiation therapy?

The INT 0139 trial reported a very high mortality in patients undergoing pneumonectomy after neoadjuvant radiation as part of trimodality therapy. The major morbidity and mortality of pneumonectomy are related to pulmonary complications: aspiration, pneumonia, acute respiratory distress syndrome.

In Toronto, Darling and colleagues[32] reviewed their results and reiterated the finding of better outcomes in patients who could be resected by lobectomy. However, in the latter part of their study, they had only 1 pneumonectomy death versus 5 in the early part. They thought that with improved postoperative care and improved technical experience they had better outcomes and survival and concluded pneumonectomy to be feasible after radiation therapy.

Many institutions have turned a critical eye to their own pneumonectomy results and the literature, and the reported mortalities range anywhere from 3% to 21% for patients undergoing pneumonectomy after chemotherapy or 3% to 26% in patients undergoing neoadjuvant chemoradiation.[35–37]

Krasna and colleagues[38] from the University of Maryland reviewed their results for patients undergoing pneumonectomy after neoadjuvant chemoradiation (61.1 Gy). Complete pathologic response was found in 55.2% of patients. Ninety-day mortality was 3.4%, and estimated 5-year disease-free survival was 48% at the time of publication. Although the study included stage IIB-IIIB patients, they clearly demonstrated that pneumonectomy can be performed safely after high-dose concurrent chemoradiation.

Weder and colleagues[39] from the University of Zurich published their mortality data after pneumonectomy in direct response to the high mortality rate published in the INT 0139 trial. Retrospective analysis of 176 pneumonectomies (35 after chemotherapy and 141 after chemoradiation with 45 Gy) showed a mortality of only 3% and overall 5-year survival of 38%. The investigators thought that with careful patient selection, preoperative staging, and postoperative care, pneumonectomy should continue to have an important role in multimodality treatment.

In summary, although many papers after the INT 0139 publication have conceded an increased risk for pneumonectomy compared with lobectomy following radiation therapy, it is also clear that this morbidity and potential mortality is at a lower rate than that described in 0139 and may be acceptable in select cases for experienced centers.

Unresolved Issues in Treating IIIA (N2) Disease: Chemotherapy

Adjuvant versus neoadjuvant prescription

Schiller and colleagues[40] in 2002 published results of the ECOG 2005 trial comparing outcomes observed in patients receiving the 4 most commonly used chemotherapy regimens to treat stage IIIB and IV lung cancer: cisplatin plus paclitaxel, cisplatin plus gemcitabine, cisplatin plus docetaxel, or carboplatin plus paclitaxel. They found no significant difference in response rate, time to progression, or survival between any of the regimens. Although they did not study stage IIIA (N2) patients specifically, the findings established the efficacy but also lack of difference between available platinum doublet regimens.

The perceived benefit of adjuvant chemo-therapy is to help eliminate microscopic circu-lating, systemic disease, and reduce distant failure. Unfortunately, no large-scale trials have been designed to study the use of adjuvant chemotherapy specifically after surgical resection for stage IIIA (N2) disease, and most of the adju-vant data come from subset analyses of large adjuvant therapy trials, including patients across disease stages.

There is a significant rate of noncompletion of adjuvant treatment in patients. Although treatment can be administered, it is not always tolerated, and studies show a rate of 31% to 50% of noncomple-tion of recommended therapy.[41] The benefit of adjuvant therapy may not be fully demonstrated in the literature because of this rate of attrition.

Most studies evaluating adjuvant chemotherapy are multistage studies, not simply focusing on N2 disease. In addition, in the studies that included postoperative radiation, the dosing, timing, and in-dications were left up to the enrolled institution without standardization, further confounding results.

Major studies evaluating adjuvant chemotherapy

Early studies showed highly variable results; half demonstrate no survival benefit and the others demonstrate some benefit to adjuvant chemotherapy. Many patients suffered from treat-ment toxicity leading to a high rate of noncomple-tion of assigned therapy. Results were also often pooled together regardless of stage (Table 3).

Given the outcomes of N2 patients in Adjuvant Navelbine International Trialist Association (ANITA), International Adjuvant Lung Cancer Trial (IALT), and Lung Adjuvant Cisplatin Evaluation (LACE) trials, patients with incidentally discovered N2 disease are routinely referred to oncology for consideration of platinum-based adjuvant chemotherapy.

Adjuvant chemotherapy for patients who have received neoadjuvant therapy

Lymph node sterilization has been consistently shown to be a prognostic indicator for superior outcome in patients receiving neoadjuvant chemotherapy. Patients with residual N2 disease have high rates of locoregional and distant fail-ure.[46] To improve the outcomes in patients with persistent N2 disease after surgery, centers have tried different approaches to treating residual dis-ease and maintaining remission.

In INT 0139, each patient received 2 cycles of consolidation chemotherapy after surgery. Unfor-tunately, only 55% of surgical patients went on to complete this therapy compared with 74% of patients in the nonsurgical arm. It is unclear how much benefit was provided to the patients with

---

Table 3
Survival benefit of adjuvant chemotherapy

Study	Stages Studied	Total Patients (N2)	Findings	Confounding Factors
ALPI[41]	I-IIIA	1209 (310)	No benefit in progression-free survival or overall survival	31% noncompliance to treatment Majority received PORT
BLT[42]	I-IIIA	381 (99)	No benefit in progression-free survival or overall survival	56 centers enrolled Did not study by individual stage No nodal sampling in 45%
IALT[43]	I-III	1867 (549)	5% increase in 5-y survival with chemotherapy Increased disease-free survival Greatest survival benefit in stage III Cisplatin used in all	148 centers
ANITA[44]	IB-IIIA	840 (325)	Absolute survival benefit 8.6% at 5 y with the addition of chemotherapy 5-y survival 42 vs 26% in stage IIIA	Noncompliance in 50% by cycle 4 Higher rate of mortality and toxicity from chemotherapy (2% compared with 0.8% in others) PORT not standardized
LACE[45]	I-IIIA	4584 (1247)	Survival benefit with platinum doublet 5.4% in stage II and III Subgroup analysis confirmed II and IIIA benefit while stage I not	Meta-analysis that included several of the aforementioned studies Higher rate of cardiovascular complications related to chemotherapy than other studies

this therapy, but certainly the lack of delivery could have lowered survival in the postsurgical patients.[25]

Amini and colleagues[47] found the addition of chemotherapy to adjuvant regimens did not improve locoregional control but did have a beneficial impact on overall survival on multivariate analysis (hazard ratio 0.425).

Targeted therapy in IIIA (N2) regimens

Complicating matters further is the demonstration in advanced disease of the efficacy of targeted agents such as erlotinib for epidermal growth factor receptor (EGFR) mutant patients and crizotinib for tumors harboring anaplastic lymphoma kinase (ALK) translocations. How these agents are to be incorporated into neoadjuvant or adjuvant treatment regimens for locally advanced disease remains to be determined. Several phase II studies are open and enrolling to address this issue for neoadjuvant erlotinib, and the National Cancer Institute–funded ALCHEMIST (Adjuvant Lung Cancer Enrichment Marker Identification and Sequencing Trial) should provide an answer in the adjuvant setting for the subgroup of patients with N2 disease.[48]

UNRESOLVED ISSUES: RADIATION
Neoadjuvant Radiation Dose

In the wake of the Fowler and colleagues[23] trial at Fox Chase Cancer Center, radiotherapy was limited to 45 Gy for subsequent trials involving patients expected to undergo surgery due to concerns of increased postoperative morbidity and mortality associated with higher doses.

Two factors led to teams challenging this notion. First, the time taken to restage patients at 45 Gy to determine whether they are a surgical candidate delays treatment in patients who are not deemed suitable for resection, and these treatment interruptions can negatively impact survival. Second, no study had ever established the optimal dose of radiation to achieve optimal mediastinal sterilization, which has been shown to impart greater overall survival.

As stated earlier in the section covering the role of surgery in multimodality treatment, there have been many trials that have demonstrated safety when operating after 60 Gy of radiation.

More Is Not Always Better

SWOG 8805[24] demonstrated neoadjuvant radiation to be safe and achieved a mediastinal nodal clearance of 50% using 45 Gy radiation.

If 45 Gy was good enough to achieve a 50% clearance, should not t more radiation be better?

The RTOG 0617 trial aimed to compare survival of patients with unresectable stage III NSCLC receiving standard-dose versus high-dose conformal radiotherapy and concurrent chemotherapy.

Over a 4-year period, 166 patients were assigned to receive standard chemoradiation (60 Gy), 121 patients were assigned to high-dose chemoradiation (74 Gy), 147 patients were assigned to standard chemoradiation and cetuximab, and 110 patients were assigned to high-dose chemoradiation and cetuximab. The patients who received 74 Gy of radiation had a higher rate of noncompliance and treatment delays and had worse survival compared with 60 Gy (20.3 months vs 28.7 months median survival). The investigators concluded that high-dose radiation may in fact be harmful to patients.[49]

There is certainly a limit to the benefits seen with neoadjuvant radiation therapy and a threshold above which patients will suffer too much toxicity. These trials provide compelling evidence to consider 60 Gy radiation as the optimal neoadjuvant regimen.

Is Neoadjuvant Radiation the Right Paradigm to Follow?

Although radiation seems to yield a higher level of mediastinal nodal sterilization than cytotoxic chemotherapy alone, not all institutions have shown this to translate into improved outcomes in disease-free survival or overall survival. In addition, there is a higher incidence of morbidity and expense with the therapy.

In 2012, the group from Duke performed a systematic review of published randomized controlled trials and retrospective reviews of multimodality management of stage IIIA (N2) disease. Seven studies were included for patients who underwent resection after treatment with induction chemotherapy alone or induction chemoradiation. The study was unable to show increased survival from adding neoadjuvant radiation to neoadjuvant chemotherapy in the treatment of N2 disease. They concluded the disadvantages of using radiation: patient morbidity such as pneumonitis and cardiac dysfunction, cost, and some reports of increased surgical complication rates, could not be justified given the lack of demonstrated survival benefit. However, because of the small numbers, additional trials are certainly warranted.[50]

Interestingly, in 2010, National Comprehensive Cancer Network member institutions were polled, and 50% reported using chemoradiation as their neoadjuvant regimen, whereas the other half reported using just chemotherapy in the treatment of stage IIIA (N2) disease.[51]

Clearly, there is no consensus among experts in the field as to the optimum treatment algorithm. All can agree that mediastinal sterilization in patients radiated neoadjuvantly seems to confer the greatest survival advantage. The challenge remains to determine the best way to achieve this without causing undue morbidity and mortality from treatments offered.

Revisiting Postoperative Radiation Therapy

The benefit of postoperative radiation therapy (PORT) in the treatment of patients who have undergone surgical resection of an N2-positive NSCLC remains unclear.

Proponents of PORT suggest that the added local control provided by radiation therapy is beneficial regardless of whether the radiation is administered preoperatively or postoperatively.

Critics suggest that PORT has not been shown to benefit patients in most studies and in some have ultimately caused harm.

The PORT meta-analysis, published initially in1998 with an update in 2005, was a systematic review of available randomized controlled studies evaluating outcomes of patients receiving postoperative radiotherapy. Eleven trials were included with more than 2000 patients. Interestingly, although patients with early stage lung cancer (N0 or N1 disease) showed worse outcome with PORT and an increased risk of death, those with N2 disease did not have increased risk of death and showed improved local control. Unfortunately, this is a retrospective review spanning several decades with outdated radiation treatment regimens, with inconsistency in timing of the delivery of radiation after surgery, and with many patients suffering significant treatment toxicity.[52]

PORT may have an important place in the treatment of stage IIIA (N2) disease in 2 areas: (1) in patients with incidentally discovered N2 disease at the time of resection; and (2) in patients undergoing neoadjuvant chemotherapy only followed by resection with persistent lymph node involvement. Several studies have found that patients who underwent chemotherapy followed by resection have a 20% to 40% local recurrence at 5 years. With modern radiation therapy, many think that a more demonstrable improvement in survival should be seen in patients receiving PORT.

Several retrospective analyses performed in the wake of PORT again confirmed improvement in local control in the setting of N2 disease, but also suggested that PORT can enhance overall survival. A Surveillance, Epidemiology, and End Results study evaluated PORT in stage II and III patients. Investigators found in the subgroup analysis that patients with N2 disease had an enhanced disease-free survival (36% vs 27%) and overall 5-year survival (27% vs 20%) in patients who received PORT.[53]

In the ANITA trial, PORT was delivered at the discretion of the treatment center. Overall, 28% of patients were treated with radiation, of whom 50% had N2 disease. Radiotherapy in this group improved survival to 47% at 5 years when combined with chemotherapy. This finding compared very favorably with 5-year survival of 34% in the adjuvant chemotherapy group and 17% in patients who received no adjuvant treatment.[44]

The largest study to date is an analysis of the National Cancer Database and included 4483 patients with N2 disease who underwent complete resection followed by sequential chemotherapy and radiation. On multivariate analysis, administration of PORT was one of the factors that predicted improved overall survival. The study reported increased 5-year survival from 34.8% to 39.3% (**Table 4**).[58]

Table 4
Postoperative radiation therapy trials

Authors	Study Population	Study Outcomes
Lally et al,[53] 2006	Stage II-III	Improved survival in patients with N2 disease
Urban et al,[54] 2013	N0-N2	Benefit to survival in patients with multistation N2 disease
Douillard et al,[55] 2008	Stage I-III	Improved survival in N2 both with and without adjuvant chemotherapy
Billiet et al,[56] 2014	Stage III	Increased time to recurrence
Kim et al,[57] 2014	Stage IIIA-N2	Improved locoregional control
Robinson et al,[58] 2015	Stage IIIA-N2	Improved overall survival
Amini et al,[47] 2012	Stage IIIA-N2	Preoperative chemotherapy, followed by surgery and radiation, is safe

The Lung Adjuvant Radiation Trial is currently accruing patients throughout multiple centers in Europe. Patients with N2 disease are being randomized to 54 Gy adjuvant radiation after complete resection. This trial will serve to better clarify the potential survival benefit in this complex subgroup of patients.[59]

Evolving Radiation Therapy

More modern techniques have reduced toxicity while improving the effectiveness of radiation delivered. Studies using these techniques have noted reduced treatment-related risk of death and no statistically significant difference in deaths from intercurrent disease.[60]

It is important to note that radiation therapy continues to evolve and improve. Planning has changed from 2-dimensional to 4-dimensional volumetric planning, guided by CT imaging; this has enabled superior tumor localization with more accurate margins and less injury to healthy surrounding tissue. Improved dosimetry and intensity modulation have allowed for more precise delivery of treatment. In addition, image-guided adaptive radiation therapy technology has begun to adapt imaging feedback of residual disease and residual physiologic activity to guide each additional treatment to the remaining active cells.[61]

THE FUTURE—MORE COMPLICATED, NOT LESS
Proton Beam Therapy

Proton beam therapy is also being trialed in centers around the United States for the treatment of NSCLC. Initial reports suggest a more limited toxicity when compared with conventional radiation therapy, facilitating higher radiation doses and improving treatment outcome.[62] No long-term data are available at this time. How best to incorporate proton therapy into multimodality treatment protocols for locally advanced NSCLC remains to be determined.

Immunotherapy

Immunotherapy is an exciting area of research in interest in the treatment of lung cancer. Immunotherapies may be broken down into 4 major groups: checkpoint inhibitors, monoclonal antibodies, therapeutic vaccines, and adoptive cell therapy. The goal with these treatments is to help generate a more vigorous immune response to lung cancer antigens, enabling the host to more effectively mount an immune attack on the tumor.

Immunotherapy is being studied as an option for more advanced stages of disease (stage IIIB and IV) and in patients whose disease progresses after first-line chemotherapy, radiation, or surgery. Phase III trials have demonstrated improved survival for checkpoint inhibitors compared with conventional treatments.[63] Several single-institution and small multi-institution studies are underway to address the role of neoadjuvant checkpoint inhibition for stage II and locally advanced NSCLC. This field is rapidly evolving with an emerging but as of yet undefined role for immunotherapy in multimodality treatment protocols.

Targeted Therapy

Cancer is a genetic disease driven by genetic mutations, and there is growing evidence that patients benefit from treatment that is tailored to the specific genetic makeup of their cancer. US Food and Drug Administration–approved targeted agents in lung cancer include erlotinib for EGFR mutant tumors, and crizotinib for those harboring ALK translocations. Despite that it is not really known how to use these existing agents in multimodality regimens for locally advanced disease, many further drugs are in development and being tested in stage IV disease. Running trials for smaller subsets of the overall population of locally advanced patients that are resectable and harbor specific, targetable mutations will be a significant challenge and may not be possible.

Feasibility trials have demonstrated safety with adding targeted therapies to multimodality regimens without an increase in morbidity and mortality. Therefore, targeted therapies have been incorporated more frequently into multimodality regimens for patients with N2 disease, where a targetable mutation exists. Although optimal timing and length of treatment remain undecided, published studies have shown favorable toxicity profile, safety with surgery, and potential benefit to overall survival.[64] The authors have some limited experience to date at Mayo Clinic for patients with locally advanced disease treated neoadjuvantly with either erlotinib or crizotinib for 8 weeks before surgery, with drug continued right up to the day before surgery and then restarted immediately following surgery when a normal diet is resumed.

SUMMARY
Evidence-based Treatment Regimens for Potentially Resectable IIIA (N2) Disease

Although at risk of inciting further controversy just by writing it down, the following can be summarized as acceptable treatment approaches in the modern era. Varying levels of evidence, from weak to level 1 evidence from randomized phase III data, exist in support of each.

1. Adjuvant chemotherapy ± adjuvant radiation for N2 disease discovered at the time of surgery (so-called occult N2 disease). It is also reasonable to back out of this scenario if minimal morbidity risk has been incurred and not resect, essentially starting over with the patient using either neoadjuvant or definitive chemoradiation treatment approaches.
2. For known N2 disease, neoadjuvant chemotherapy followed by surgical resection, +/− adjuvant chemotherapy and/or adjuvant radiation.
3. For known N2 disease, neoadjuvant chemoradiation using 45 to 60 Gy, followed by surgical resection.

This list is by no means comprehensive and leaves many gaps for specific patient scenarios.

What Can Be Said Definitively from the Literature?

- The extent of N2 disease can vary dramatically and correlates with survival.
- Mediastinal sterilization with neoadjuvant chemoradiation confers a superior 5-year survival with surgical resection, emphasizing the importance of preoperative treatment while maintaining acceptable levels of toxicity.
- A lobectomy is safer than a pneumonectomy following neoadjuvant chemoradiation.
- Surgery can be performed safely after neoadjuvant chemoradiation.

Unfortunately, many controversies still remain within the field, with a paucity of clinical trials dedicated to the specific study of N2 disease. Although studies exist that are currently enrolling patients with the goal of providing clarity to many of these issues, the majority will remain unresolved for the foreseeable future and lay in the subjective hands of expert opinion and consensus guidelines.

Ongoing Challenges in Studying Stage IIIA (N2) Disease

Large, prospective, randomized trials studying stage IIIA (N2) disease are needed to help better define optimal treatment for these patients. However, it is very difficult to accomplish large-scale trials in this setting given the limited number of potentially resectable IIIA (N2) patients. With the rapid development of novel therapies, be it new targeted agents, immunotherapy, or novel radiation therapy approaches, many new regimens of the day are obsolete by the time clinical trials can be designed and accrued to.

In this context, novel clinical trial designs are clearly necessary to study best treatment approaches for locally advanced IIIA (N2) disease. Traditional phase 1, 2, and 3 clinical trial structures are impractical, take too long to complete, and can be obsolete by the time they are completed. Novel designs such as adaptive, basket, and umbrella trial designs offer opportunity for the science of clinical trials to keep up with advances in the field.

Final Statement

There is no consensus as to the optimal management of IIIA (N2) NSCLC, nor for the role of surgery in treating this disease stage. Clinical trial evidence struggles to keep up with technology advancement and the evolution of expert opinion. Further developments in both will stimulate and maintain controversy in the field for years to come.

REFERENCES

1. Surveillance, epidemiology and end results. Bethesda (MD): US National Institutes of Health National Cancer Institute; 2010.
2. Silvestri GA, Gonzalez AV, Jantz MA, et al. Methods for staging non-small cell lung cancer: diagnosis and management of lung cancer, 3rd ed: American College of Chest Physicians evidence-based clinical practice guidelines. Chest 2013;143(5):211S–50S.
3. Yasafuku K, Pierre A, Darling G, et al. A prospective controlled trial of endobronchial ultrasound-guided transbronchial needle aspiration compared with mediastinoscopy for mediastinal lymph node staging of lung cancer. Presented at the 91st Annual Meeting of the American Association for Thoracic Surgery. Philadelphia, May 7–11, 2011.
4. Wigle DA. The beginning of the end for mediastinoscopy. J Thorac Oncol 2008;3(6):561–2.
5. Darling GE, Dickie AJ, Malthaner RA, et al. Invasive mediastinal staging of non-small-cell lung cancer: a clinical practice guideline. Curr Oncol 2011;18(6):e304–10.
6. Lee PC, Port JL, Korst RJ, et al. Risk factors for occult mediastinal metastases in clinical stage I non-small cell lung cancer. Ann Thorac Surg 2007;84(1):177–81.
7. Al-Sarraf N, Aziz R, Gately K, et al. Pattern and predictors of occult mediastinal lymph node involvement in non-small cell lung cancer patients with negative mediastinal update on positron emission tomography. Eur J Cardiothorac Surg 2008;33(1):104–9.
8. Jiang L, Jiang S, Lin Y, et al. Nomogram to predict occult N2 lymph nodes metastases in patients with

squamous non-small cell lung cancer. Medicine 2015;94(46):e2054.

9. Defranchi SA, Cassivi SD, Nichols FC, et al. N2 disease in T1 non-small cell lung cancer. Ann Thorac Surg 2009;88(3):924–8.

10. Veeramachaneni NK, Feins RH, Stephenson BJK, et al. Management of stage IIIA non-small cell lung cancer by thoracic surgeons in North America. Ann Thorac Surg 2012;94(3):922–8.

11. Louie BE, Kapur S, Farivar AS, et al. Safety and utility of mediastinoscopy in non-small cell lung cancer in a complex mediastinum. Ann Thorac Surg 2011; 92:278–83.

12. Cerfolio RJ, Bryant AS, Ojha B. Restaging patients with N2 (stage IIIA) non-small cell lung cancer after neoadjuvant chemoradiotherapy: a prospective study. J Thorac Cardiovasc Surg 2006;131(6): 1229–35.

13. Machtay M, Hsy C, Komaki R, et al. Effect of overall treatment time on outcomes after concurrent chemoradiation for locally advanced non-small-cell lung carcinoma: analysis of the Radiation Therapy Oncology Group (RTOG) experience. Int J Radiat Oncol Biol Phys 2005;63:667–71.

14. Pijls Johannesma M, Houben R, Boersma L, et al. High-dose radiotherapy or concurrent chemoradiation in lung cancer patients only induces a temporary, reversible decline in QoL. Radiother Oncol 2009;91:443–8.

15. Minami-Shimmyo Y, Ohe Y, Yamamoto S, et al. Risk factors for treatment-related death associated with chemotherapy and thoracic radiotherapy for lung cancer. J Thorac Oncol 2012;7(10):177–82.

16. Rosell R, Gomez-Codina J, Camps C, et al. A randomized trial comparing preoperative chemotherapy plus surgery with surgery alone in patients with non-small cell lung cancer. N Engl J Med 1994;330(3):153–8.

17. Roth J, Fossella F, Komaki R, et al. A randomized trial comparing perioperative chemotherapy and surgery with surgery alone in resectable stage IIIA non-small-cell lung cancer. J Natl Cancer Inst 1994;86(9):673–80.

18. Pisters KM, Vallteres E, Bunn P, et al, Southwest Oncology Group. S 9900: surgery alone or surgery plus induction paclitaxel carboplatin (PC) chemotherapy in early stage non-small cell lung cancer (NSCLC): follow up on a phase II trial [meeting abstracts]. Clin Oncol 2007;25(18):S7521.

19. Depierre A, Milleron B, Moro-Sibilot D. Pre-operative chemotherapy followed by surgery compared with primary surgery in resectable stage I (except T1N0), II and IIIA non-small-cell lung cancer. J Clin Oncol 2002;20(1):247–53.

20. Gilligan D, Nicolson M, Smith I, et al. Pre-operative chemotherapy in patients with resectable non-small cell lung cancer: results of the MRC LU22/NVALT 2/EORTC 08012 multicentre randomised trial and update of systematic review. Lancet 2007;369(9577):1929–37.

21. Jeremic B, Shibamoto Y, Acimovic L, et al. Hyperfractionated radiation therapy with or without concurrent low-dose daily carboplatin/etoposide for stage III non-small-cell lung cancer: a randomized study. J Clin Oncol 1996;14(4):1065–70.

22. Schaakekoning C, Vandenbogaert W, Dalesio O, et al. Effects of concomitant cisplatin and radiotherapy on inoperable non-small-cell lung cancer. N Engl J Med 1992;326(8):524–30.

23. Fowler WC, Langer CJ, Curran WJ, et al. Postoperative complications after combined neoadjuvant treatment of lung cancer. Ann Thorac Surg 1993; 55(4):986–9.

24. Albain K, Rusch V, Crowley J, et al. Long term survival after concurrent cisplatin/etoposide (PE) plus chest radiotherapy (RT) followed by surgery in bulky, stages IIIA (N2) and IIIB non-small cell lung cancer (NSCLC): 6 year outcomes from Southwest Oncology Group Lung Committee 8805. Clin Oncol 1995;18:467a.

25. Albain KS, Swann RS, Rusch VW, et al. Radiotherapy plus chemotherapy with or without surgical resection for stage III non-small-cell lung cancer: a phase III randomised controlled trial. Lancet 2009; 374:379–86.

26. Andre F, Grunenwald D, Pignon JP, et al. Survival of patients with resected N2 non-small-cell lung cancer: evidence for a subclassification and implications. J Clin Oncol 2000;18(16):2981–9.

27. Suntharalingam M, Paulus R, Edelman MJ, et al. Radiation therapy oncology group protocol 02-29: a phase II trial of neoadjuvant therapy with concurrent chemotherapy and full-dose radiation therapy followed by surgical resection and consolidative therapy for locally advanced non-small cell carcinoma of the lung. Int J Radiat Oncol Biol Phys 2012;84(2):456–63.

28. Seder CW, Allen MS, Cassivi SD, et al. Stage IIIA non-small cell lung cancer: morbidity and mortality of 3 distinct multimodality regimens. Ann Thorac Surg 2013;95:1708–16.

29. Cerfolio RJ, Bryant AS, Jones VL, et al. Pulmonary resection after concurrent chemotherapy and high dose (60Gy) radiation for non small-cell lung cancer is safe and may provide increased survival. Eur J Cardiothorac Surg 2009;35:718–23.

30. Van Meerbeeck JP, Kramer GWPM, Van Schil PEY, et al, on behalf of the EORTC. Randomized controlled trial of resection versus radiotherapy after induction chemotherapy in stage IIIA-N2 non-small-cell lung cancer. J Natl Cancer Inst 2007;99(6): 442–50.

31. Cerfolio RJ, Maniscalco L, Bryant AS. The treatment of patients with stage IIIA non-small cell lung cancer

from N2 disease: who returns to the surgical arena and who survives. Ann Thorac Surg 2008;86(3):912–20.

32. Darling GE, Li F, Patsios D, et al. Neoadjuvant chemoradiation and surgery improves survival outcomes compared with definitive chemoradiation in the treatment of stage IIIA N2 non-small-cell lung cancer. Eur J Cardiothorac Surg 2015;48(5):684–90.

33. Myers BF, Haddad R, Siegel BA, et al. Cost-effectiveness of routine mediastinoscopy in computer tomography- and positron emission tomography-screened patients with stage I lung cancer. J Thorac Cardiovasc Surg 2006;131(4):822–9.

34. Darling GE, Allen MS, Decker PA, et al. Randomized trial of mediastinal lymph node sampling versus complete lymphadenectomy during pulmonary resection in the patient with N0 or N1 (less than hilar) non-small cell carcinoma: results of the American College of Surgery Oncology Group Z0030 Trial. J Thorac Cardiovasc Surg 2011;141(3):662–70.

35. Daly BD, Fernando HC, Ketchedjian A, et al. Pneumonectomy after high-dose radiation and concurrent chemotherapy for nonsmall cell lung cancer. Ann Thorac Surg 2006;82(1):227–31.

36. Allen AM, Mentzer SJ, Yeap BY, et al. Pneumonectomy after chemoradiation: the Dana-Farber Cancer Institute/Brigham and Women's Hospital experience. Cancer 2008;112(5):1106–13.

37. D'Amato TA, Ashrafi AS, Schuchert MJ, et al. Risk of pneumonectomy after induction therapy for locally advanced non-small cell lung cancer. Ann Thorac Surg 2009;88(4):1079–85.

38. Krasna MJ, Gamliel Z, Burrows WM, et al. Pneumonectomy for lung cancer after preoperative concurrent chemotherapy and high-dose radiation. Ann Thorac Surg 2010;89(1):200–6.

39. Weder W, Collard S, Eberhardt WEE, et al. Pneumonectomy is a valuable treatment option after neoadjuvant therapy for stage III non-small-cell lung cancer. J Thorac Cardiovasc Surg 2010;139(6):1424–30.

40. Schiller J, Harrington D, Belani CP, et al. Comparison of four chemotherapy regimens for advanced non-small-cell lung cancer. N Engl J Med 2002;346:92–8.

41. Scagliotti GV, Fossati R, Torri V, et al. Randomized study of adjuvant chemotherapy for completely resected stage I, II, or IIIA non-small-cell lung cancer. J Natl Cancer Inst 2003;95(19):1453–61.

42. Waller D, Peake MD, Stephens RJ, et al. Chemotherapy for patients with non-small-cell lung cancer: the surgical setting of the big lung trial. Eur J Cardiothorac Surg 2004;26(1):173–82.

43. NSCLC Meta-analyses Collaborative Group. Adjuvant chemotherapy, with or without postoperative radiotherapy, in operable non-small-cell lung cancer: two meta-analyses of individual patient data. Lancet 2010;375(9722):1267–77.

44. Douillard JY, Rosell R, De Lena M, et al. Adjuvant vinorelbine plus cisplatin vs. observation in patients with completely resected stage IB-IIIA non-small-cell lung cancer (Adjuvant Navelbine International Trialist Association [ANITA]): a randomized controlled trial. Lancet Oncol 2006;7:719–27.

45. Pignon JP, Tribodet H, Scagliotti GV, et al. Lung adjuvant cisplatin evaluation: a pooled analysis by the LACE Collaborative Group. J Clin Oncol 2008;26(21):3552–9.

46. Jaklitsch MT, Herndon JE, Decamp MM, et al. Nodal downstaging predicts survival following induction chemotherapy for stage IIIA (N2) non-small cell lung cancer in CALGB Protocol #8935. J Surg Oncol 2006;94:599–606.

47. Amini A, Correa AM, Komaki R, et al. The role of consolidation therapy for stage III non-small cell lung cancer with persistent N2 disease after induction chemotherapy. Ann Thorac Surg 2012;94(3):914–20.

48. Oxnard GR, Watt C, Wigle D, et al. Biomarker-driven adjuvant targeted therapy for NSCLC—the ALCHEMIST trials. Bull Am Coll Surg 2015;100(9):25–7.

49. Bradley JD, Paulus R, Komaki R, et al. Standard-dose versus high-dose conformal radiotherapy with concurrent and consolidation carboplatin plus paclitaxel with or without cetuximab for patients with stage IIIA or IIIB non-small-cell lung cancer (RTOG 0617): a randomised, two-by-two factorial phase 3 study. Lancet Oncol 2015;16(2):187–99.

50. Shah AA, Berry MF, Tzao C, et al. Induction chemoradiation is not superior to induction chemotherapy alone in stage IIIA lung cancer. Ann Thorac Surg 2012;93:1807.

51. NCCN clinical practice guidelines in oncology: non-small cell lung cancer. Available at: https://www.nccn.org/professionals/physician_gls/pdf/nscl.pdf. Accessed November 15, 2015.

52. PORT Meta-Analysis Trialist Group. Postoperative radiotherapy for non-small cell lung cancer. Cochrane Database Syst Rev 2000;(2):CD002142.

53. Lally BE, Zelterman D, Colasanto JM, et al. Postoperative radiotherapy for stage II or III non-small-cell lung cancer using the surveillance, epidemiology, and end results database. J Clin Oncol 2006;24(19):2998–3006.

54. Urban D, Bar J, Solomon B, et al. Lymph node ratio may predict the benefit of postoperative radiotherapy in non-small-cell lung cancer. J Thorac Oncol 2013;8(7):940–6.

55. Douillard JY, Rosell R, DeLena M, et al. Impact of postoperative radiation therapy on survival in patients with complete resection and stage I, II, or IIIA non-small-cell lung cancer treated with adjuvant chemotherapy: the Adjuvant Navelbine International Trialist Association (ANITA) Randomized Trial. Int J Radiat Oncol Biol Phys 2008;72(3):695–701.

56. Billiet C, Decaluwé H, Peeters S, et al. Modern postoperative radiotherapy for stage III non-small cell lung cancer may improve local control and survival: a meta-analysis. Radiother Oncol 2014;110(1):3–8.

57. Kim BH, Kim HJ, Wu HG, et al. Role of postoperative radiotherapy after curative resection and adjuvant chemotherapy for patients with pathological stage N2 non-small-cell lung cancer: a propensity score matching analysis. Clin Lung Cancer 2014;15(5): 356–64.

58. Robinson CG, Patel AP, Bradley JD, et al. Postoperative radiotherapy for pathologic N2 non-small-cell lung cancer treated with adjuvant chemotherapy: a review of the National Cancer Data Base. J Clin Oncol 2015;33(8):870–6.

59. Le Péchoux C. Role of postoperative radiotherapy in resected non-small cell lung cancer: a reassessment based on new data. Oncologist 2011;16(5): 672–81.

60. Wakelee HA, Stephenson P, Keller SM, et al. Postoperative radiotherapy (PORT) or chemoradiotherapy (CPORT) following resection of stages II and IIIA non-small cell lung cancer (NSCLC) does not increase the expected risk of death from intercurrent disease (DID) in Eastern Cooperative Oncology Group (ECOG) trial E3590. Lung Cancer 2005; 48(3):389–97.

61. Glide-Hurst CK, Chetty IJ. Improving radiotherapy planning, delivery, accuracy and normal tissue sparing using cutting edge technologies. J Thorac Dis 2014;6(4):303–18.

62. Sejpal S, Komaki R, Tsao A, et al. Early findings on toxicity of proton beam therapy with concurrent chemotherapy for nonsmall cell lung cancer. Cancer 2011;117(13):3004–13.

63. Borghaei H, Pas-Ares L, Horn L, et al. Nivolumab versus docetaxel in advanced nonsquamous non-small-cell lung cancer. N Engl J Med 2015;373: 1627–39.

64. Ratto GB, Costa R, Maineri P, et al. Neo-adjuvant chemo/immunotherapy in the treatment of stage III (N2) non-small cell lung cancer: a phase I/II pilot study. Int J Immunopathol Pharmacol 2011;24(4): 1005–16.

Surgical Management of Oligometastatic Non–Small Cell Lung Cancer

Michael Lanuti, MD

KEYWORDS

- Oligometastases • Metastases • Non–small lung cancer • Surgery • Metastectomy

KEY POINTS

- Pulmonary resection of primary lung cancer and the oligometastatic site should only be considered in patients with good performance status and adequate lung function.
- Despite the absence of anatomically enlarged or fludeoxyglucose-negative mediastinal lymph nodes, invasive mediastinal staging with endobronchial ultrasound or mediastinoscopy is recommended in patients being considered for a curative approach to oligometastatic non–small cell lung cancer (NSCLC).
- Intrathoracic lymph node disease (N1, N2, N3) is associated with worse outcome in oligometastatic NSCLC.
- Primary lung cancer with synchronous solitary cranial or adrenal metastases should be evaluated for curative aggressive local therapy.
- Curative intent for oligometastatic disease to organs other than lung, brain, adrenal should be considered on a case-by-case basis.

INTRODUCTION

Selecting patients with M1a-b non–small cell lung cancer (NSCLC) for curative treatment is controversial and challenging. Five-year survival in stage IV NSCLC remains as low as 1% with median survival of 8 to 11 months.[1] Tumor genotyping and the implementation of targeted chemotherapy have transformed the management of metastatic NSCLC resulting in prolonged survival in a subgroup of patients.[2] There is another subgroup of patients with stage IV NSCLC who present with a primary lung cancer and a single site of extrapulmonary oligometastatic disease that seem to benefit from complete resection or local control of all disease. Systematic review of the literature reporting on 2176 patients who harbor 1 to 3 metastases of NSCLC treated with surgical metastectomy revealed a wide range of survival (median overall 5-year survival 6–52 months).[3] The most common sites of extrathoracic disease are bone, brain, adrenal, liver, and lymph node. Isolated metastases to the contralateral lung can occur, but reconciling metastatic disease versus a synchronous primary lung cancer is often challenging despite tumor genotyping. Analysis of variables has demonstrated unfavorable post-recurrence outcomes with non-adenocarcinoma histology, short disease interval, polymetastases, older age, and the presence of liver or bone metastasis.[3] Observations of survival in this patient subgroup are still subject to scrutiny because

Disclosure Statement: There are no commercial or financial conflicts. There are no funding sources.
Division of Thoracic Surgery, Harvard Medical School, Massachusetts General Hospital, 55 Fruit Street, Blake 1570, Boston, MA 02114, USA
E-mail address: MLanuti@mgh.harvard.edu

Thorac Surg Clin 26 (2016) 287–294
http://dx.doi.org/10.1016/j.thorsurg.2016.04.002

treatment intervention versus favorable tumor biology cannot be easily distinguished.

DEFINITION OF OLIGOMETASTATIC DISEASE

The term *oligometastases* is synonymous with isolated distant metastases but was originally introduced by Hellman and Weichselbaum[4] in 1995 to describe a state of limited systemic metastatic disease whereby local therapies could be curative.[5] The concept of an "oligometastatic state" represents a less biologically aggressive neoplasm whereby the number of metastatic sites (usually single) and location (limited to a single organ) remains stable over time. The term has morphed into including more than one site of metastatic disease in a single organ (ie, 1–3 brain metastases). It should also be mentioned that the classic interpretation of oligometastatic lung cancer includes *synchronous* presentation of a primary tumor (in this case NSCLC) and a distant site of extrapulmonary disease. The development of *metachronous* disease involving a single organ site sometime after treatment of the primary tumor can also be termed an oligometastatic state. Metachronous disease is often defined as a newly recognized site of oligometastatic disease at a time interval of 3 or more months from the time of treatment. Curative surgery or local control of metastatic disease is primarily reserved for M1b disease. The M descriptor in the seventh edition of TNM staging of NSCLC includes M1a (separate tumor nodules in a contralateral lobe, tumor with associated pleural nodules, malignant pleural effusion, or pericardial effusion) and M1b (extrathoracic metastases).[6] Median survival for M1a and M1b disease is 11.5 and 7.5 months, respectively. In the proposed eighth edition of TNM staging, the M descriptor will be reclassified as M1a, M1b (single metastatic lesion in one organ), and M1c (multiple metastases in either single organ or multiple organs). Patients with single extrathoracic metastasis had better prognosis than those with multiple metastatic lesions in one organ or multiple organs involved (new M1c).[7,8]

PRINCIPLES OF SURGICAL TREATMENT

When considering surgery in the treatment of oligometastatic NSCLC, a careful investigation into the presence of intrathoracic nodal metastases is mandatory. Despite negative mediastinal lymph nodes on staging computed tomography (CT)–PET, invasive mediastinal staging with endobronchial ultrasound or mediastinoscopy is highly recommended in this high-risk population. Patients who demonstrate pathologic N1 or N2

disease often do not derive long-term survival from removing the primary tumor and oligometastatic site.[9] The primary tumor should be amenable to complete R0 resection; anything less would argue against a curative approach to oligometastatic disease. Oligometastatic disease sites should be amenable to aggressive complete local control either by surgery or by an ablative modality, such as stereotactic radiosurgery (SRS) for brain metastases or stereotactic body radiotherapy (SBRT).

There is no consensus on how and when to institute systemic chemotherapy in relation to local control of either the oligometastatic site or the primary. In a retrospective series[10] of 53 patients at a single center where 85% harbored a single synchronous site of metastatic disease, 4 different approaches were described: (1) local control of the oligometastatic site followed by neoadjuvant chemotherapy then lung surgery, (2) local control of the oligometastatic site followed by lung surgery, (3) induction chemotherapy followed by lung surgery and then local control of the oligometastatic site, and finally (4) lung surgery and treatment of the oligometastatic site simultaneously. The investigators concluded that there is no advantage to any particular sequence of therapy. Predictors of favorable outcome included single site of disease diagnosed by CT-PET, absence of weight loss greater than 10%, complete resection, and pathologic N0 disease. Although extended survival can be achieved in a subgroup of patients, a high proportion of patients with oligometastatic NSCLC fail locally and systemically soon after treatment, with a median time to recurrence of 12 months.

Prospective evaluation of oligometastatic disease in NSCLC has only been reported in 2 published single-center series. A phase II trial of chemotherapy and surgery for patients with oligometastatic NSCLC was undertaken in 23 patients with a solitary synchronous M1 site.[11] Nearly 50% of the patients harbored N2 disease, and the oligometastatic site was intracranial in 14 patients. Patients received 3 cycles of chemotherapy (cisplatin, mitomycin, vinblastine) followed by resection of all disease sites and then 2 cycles of outback chemotherapy. Median survival was 11 months, and the investigators concluded that induction chemotherapy was difficult to complete and survival did not seem superior to the historical experience of surgery alone. In a separate phase II single-arm study, 39 patients with stage IV NSCLC and less than 5 synchronous metastatic lesions underwent radical local treatment of all sites (including the primary) with either surgery or radiotherapy.[12] The most common sites of M1 disease were brain (44%), bone (18%), and adrenal gland

(10%). Most patients (87%) were diagnosed with a single distant metastasis. Median progression-free survival was 10.2 months for adrenal locations, 13.5 months for bone, and 13.6 months for brain. Fifteen percent of patients did not show progression after 2 years prompting the investigators to conclude that a subgroup of patients may be cured with a strategy of radical local control in the absence of systemic therapy.

ORGAN-SPECIFIC CONSIDERATIONS

Plönes and colleagues[13] reported survival differences based on metastatic site of origin with 23.4 months for patients with soft tissue metastasis, 16.7 months for patients with brain metastasis, 9.5 months for patients with adrenal gland involvement, and only 4.3 months for patients with bone metastasis ($P < 0.005$). Other sites of rare metastatic deposits include breast, pancreas,[14] pectoralis muscle,[15] and small bowel. Luketich and colleagues[16] reported on long-term survivors who presented with *metachronous* oligometastatic disease (median interval 19.5 [range 5–71 months]) after lobectomy with single sites of extracranial and extra-adrenal metastases. The 10-year actuarial survival for this series of

14 patients was 86% at a median follow-up of 101 months.

Solitary Brain Metastasis

Much controversy surrounds the appropriate management of primary lung cancer in patients with synchronous intracranial metastases. Intracranial metastases are found in 25% to 35% of patients who present with a new diagnosis of NSCLC. Pathologic survey of autopsy series published in 1954 demonstrated cerebral metastases in 53% of patients with a diagnosis of lung cancer.[17] Historically, whole-brain radiation alone was offered as first-line therapy for the management of intracranial metastases with median survival of 3 to 6 months. Several retrospective single-center case series have reported long-term survival in a subgroup of patients with solitary brain metastases who underwent aggressive treatment of both the brain metastases and the locoregional disease in the lung (**Table 1**).[18–24] In these series, the 5-year survival for patients who underwent complete resection averages 21% (range, 1–35), with treatment-related mortality of 2%. The Mayo Clinic reported on a series of 28 patients whereby 5-year survival in resected patients with node negative (N0) NSCLC and synchronous brain

Table 1
Review of the literature in published series with synchronous oligometastatic lung cancer to brain

Series	N	Complete Resection (%)	Nodal Stage (No. of Patients)	Mortality (%)	Survival Influenced by TNM Stage	Survival 5-y (%)	Median
Getman et al,[18] 2004	16	87.5	N1 (3) N2 (5)	0	No squamous histology	19	8.5 mo
Billing et al,[19] 2001	28	100	N1 (5) N2 (6)	0	Yes	21 35 (N0)	24 mo
Bonnette et al,[20] 2001	103	92	N1 (23) N2 (35)	2	No	11	12 mo
Mussi et al,[21] 1996	19	79	N0 (8) N1/2 (7)	—	Yes	6.6	18 mo
Burt et al,[22] 1992	65	78	N0 (27) N2 (30)	—	No	16	21 mo
Rossi et al,[23] 1987	40	100	N0 (15) N1 (15) N2 (10)	1.5	Yes	12.5 20 (N0)	24 mo
Magilligan et al,[24] 1986	14	—	—	2	No	21	—

Dash indicates data not reported.
Abbreviation: TNM, tumor-node-metastasis.

metastases was far superior compared with the presence of N1/N2 disease (median survival 44 vs 10 months, respectively).[19] No patient with lymph node metastases survived longer than 3 years after resection.

Selection of appropriate candidates for this curative treatment of oligometastatic NSCLC requires precise staging by means of diagnostic imaging, including the use of PET-CT, brain MRI, and invasive mediastinal staging. Candidates must have sufficient cardiopulmonary reserve and ideally harbor a limited number ($\leq$3) of intracranial metastases. Others have corroborated that patients with intrathoracic nodal metastases (N1 or N2) often have a relapse after aggressive therapy, with a reported overall survival (OS) of less than 3 years.[25]

Before surgical staging and resection of the primary tumor, patients with *symptomatic* brain metastases should *first* undergo craniotomy and resection or stereotactic radiosurgery, with or without whole-brain radiation therapy (WBRT) to prevent neurologic sequelae. Although not specific for NSCLC histology, the study by Patchell and colleagues,[26] which randomized patients with a single brain metastasis to WBRT alone versus surgical resection plus WBRT, found a survival benefit in those who received surgery. Surgical resection followed by WBRT is thought to be a better treatment than surgical resection alone by virtue of improved local control of the tumor bed and in the brain overall.[27] For tumors that are less than 3 cm in diameter and that may be surgically inaccessible, SRS without WBRT can confer virtually the same survival rate as surgery.[28] These approaches are associated with a 0% to 3% mortality rate.

The American College of Chest Physicians (ACCP) sponsored an evidence-based review of lung cancer treatment (last updated in 2013)[29] that recommends

- In patients with an isolated brain metastasis from NSCLC being considered for curative treatment, invasive mediastinal staging and extrathoracic imaging (either whole-body PET or abdominal CT plus bone scan) are suggested.
- Resection or radiosurgical ablation of an isolated brain metastasis in patients with no other sites of metastases and a *synchronous* resectable N0, N1 primary NSCLC is recommended. The National Cancer Care Network (NCCN) endorsed this paradigm in version 6 of 2015 but also recognized the use of SBRT for control of the primary lung cancer if surgical candidacy was poor.[30]

- In patients with no other sites of metastases and a previously completely resected primary NSCLC (*metachronous* presentation), resection or radiosurgical ablation of an isolated brain metastasis is recommended.

Factors that seem to influence improvement in survival include complete (R0) lung resection, low T stage and N status, short interval between pulmonary resection and craniotomy/SRS, number of brain lesions ($\leq$3), metachronous presentation, and supratentorial location.

Solitary Adrenal Metastases

The adrenal gland is a common site of metastatic NSCLC. Detection of a single adrenal metastasis is less frequent than brain, with an incidence of 1.6% to 4.0% of resectable NSCLCs.[31] Adrenal enlargement during the staging of NSCLC does not necessarily indicate metastatic disease because the prevalence of adrenal incidentalomas is 4% to 5% in radiologic series where many (>80%) are benign.[32] Although PET-CT and adrenal protocol CT can be very helpful to distinguish metastatic disease, histopathologic confirmation of indeterminate adrenal nodules should be obtained before lung cancer surgery.[33] There are no randomized data on the treatment of synchronous or metachronous oligometastatic NSCLC involving the adrenal gland. Multiple small retrospective series (depicted in **Table 2**) report on outcomes of NSCLC with oligometastatic disease to the adrenal gland.[34–41] Pooled analysis of outcomes from adrenalectomy (n = 114) for isolated adrenal metastases from NSCLC in multiple (n = 10) published series[42] revealed shorter median OS for synchronous versus metachronous disease (12 vs 31 months, P = .02). Importantly, 5-year OS estimates were equivalent at 25% in both groups. The investigators concluded that adrenalectomy should be considered as a therapeutic option in patients with NSCLC for either synchronous or metachronous adrenal metastasis.

In a retrospective series of 37 highly selected patients with NSCLC and isolated adrenal metastases (20 patients underwent adrenalectomy and the remainder were treated nonoperatively), laterality and the presence of mediastinal lymph node disease were significant.[37] Those patients with pathologic N1 or N0 disease had a 5-year OS of 52%, whereas no patient with N2 disease survived 5 years (P = .008). The investigators also noted that patients with ipsilateral disease had a 5-year survival of 83% compared with 0% for patients with contralateral adrenal metastases (P = .003). This phenomenon of improved OS in ipsilateral adrenal metastases was also observed in a more

Table 2
Outcomes of oligometastatic non–small cell lung cancer with adrenal site of disease

Series	N	Lung Cancer (%)	5-y Survival (%)	Prognostic Factors
Tanvetyanon et al,[42] 2008	110	100	25	None
Pham et al,[34] 2001	78	100	40	Negative intrathoracic nodes
Porte et al,[35] 2001	43	100	12	None
Mercier et al,[36] 2005	23	100	23	DFI >6 mo
Raz et al,[37] 2011	20	100	34	Ipsilateral metastasis, N2 negative
Lucchi et al,[38] 2005	14	100	36	None
Howell et al,[39] 2013	62	50	27	DFI >12 mo, metachronous disease
Strong et al,[40] 2007	94	39	29	None
Wade et al,[41] 1998	47	30	26	None

Abbreviation: DFI, disease-free interval.

recent retrospective series of 18 patients with oligometastatic NSCLC.[43] Anatomic studies demonstrating the presence of direct retroperitoneal lymphatic channels between the chest and the adrenal gland suggest that some adrenal gland metastases may represent locoregional spread rather than hematogenous metastasis.[44]

In an evidenced-base review of NSCLC, the ACCP published guidelines for oligometastatic adrenal metastases.[29]

- In patients with an isolated adrenal metastasis from NSCLC being considered for curative-intent surgical resection, invasive mediastinal staging and extrathoracic imaging (head CT/MRI plus either whole-body PET or abdominal CT plus bone scan) are suggested.
- In patients with a *synchronous* resectable N0, N1 primary NSCLC and an isolated adrenal metastasis with no other sites of metastases, resection of the primary tumor and the adrenal metastasis is recommended. *The NCCN endorsed this paradigm in version 6 of 2015.*[30]
- In patients who have undergone a curative resection of an isolated adrenal metastasis, adjuvant chemotherapy is suggested.

There is no consensus on the therapeutic sequence of primary pulmonary resection for stage IV NSCLC and adrenalectomy. Options include pulmonary resection followed by open or laparoscopic adrenalectomy ± systemic chemotherapy versus simultaneous resection of both the lung primary and adrenal metastasis ± systemic chemotherapy. If the lung cancer is ipsilateral to the M1 site of adrenal metastasis, simultaneous resection is more appealing, where the adrenalectomy can be achieved through the ipsilateral diaphragm or via a retroperitoneal approach.

Other Organs

There is a paucity of published data on observations and outcomes of oligometastatic NSCLC to bone, liver, pancreas, breast, kidney, and intestine. A systematic review of oligometastatic NSCLC to the pancreas from which data on 32 patients were collected, curative intent resection (distal pancreatectomy or pancreaticoduodenectomy) was associated with a 5-year survival of 21%.[45]

OUTCOMES

When examining survival results in published literature of patients with oligometastatic NSCLC, there is inherent bias because patients who undergo curative strategies are highly selected. Most surgical series reporting on patients with oligometastatic NSCLC have focused on brain or adrenal metastases with very few reporting on extrapulmonary and extra-adrenal sites. Ashworth and colleagues[3] completed a systematic review of the literature focusing on 49 publications (N = 2176) inclusive of patients with NSCLC with 1 to 5 metastases treated with surgical metastectomy or an ablative radiotherapy modality (SRS or SBRT). Brain metastases were the only site of oligometastatic disease in 1236 patients, and adenocarcinoma was the most commonly observed histology. Patients with mixed metastatic sites had the longest median survival. In contrast to other published series, adrenal metastases were associated with the shortest median survivals. Control of the primary was associated with improved survival in patients with brain metastases. Multivariate analysis showed that prognostic factors for survival were control of primary tumor, N stage, and disease-free interval of more than 6 to 12 months.[3]

Systemic review of the literature from 1985 to 2012 was undertaken by Ashworth and colleagues[46] to render a meta-analysis of outcomes in the treatment of oligometastatic NSCLC. Data were obtained from centers in Europe, Asia, North America, and Australia on 757 patients with 1 to 5 synchronous or metachronous (diagnosed ≥2 months after the primary tumor) metastases treated with surgical metastectomy, SBRT, or radical external beam radiotherapy including curative treatment of the lung primary. **Table 3** depicts a summary of the location of oligometastases. Most patients (88%) harbored one site of metastatic disease whereby 52% were node negative (N0). Surgical resection was the primary modality of treatment of the lung primary in 84% of patients and for 52% of the oligometastatic sites. Five-year OS in the entire cohort was 29.4% with a median follow-up of 53 months. During the follow-up period 70% of patients progressed either locally or systemically with a median time to progression of 11 months. The longest survivals were observed in patients with metachronous metastases (5-year OS 48%). Patients with synchronous metastases and N0 status had a 5-year OS of 36%. The least favorable patient group presented with synchronous metastases and N1/N2 disease with a 5-year OS of 14%.

An attempt at examining prospective outcomes in patients with limited oligometastatic NSCLC were explored in 2 randomized phase II trials. One study, NCT00887315, randomized patients with NSCLC and 5 or less metastases (with stable disease after 2 cycles of chemotherapy) to high-dose radiotherapy to all sites of disease versus 2 additional cycles of chemotherapy. The second study, NCT00776100, randomized patients with 3 or less oligometastases (with stable disease after 2–6 cycles of chemotherapy) to observation or high-dose radiotherapy to all sites of disease. Both trials were closed because of poor accrual.

There are a few phase II clinical trials studying the efficacy of ablative treatments in oligometastatic NSCLC. The Stereotactic Ablative Radiotherapy for Comprehensive Treatment of Metastatic Tumors (SABR-COMET) trial (NCT01446744) is randomizing approximately 99 patients with primary tumors of varying histologies (up to 5 metachronous sites) to stereotactic ablative radiotherapy of all oligometastatic sites versus palliative chemotherapy and/or radiation.[47] The United Kingdom is sponsoring a phase III randomized trial (NCT02417662) examining the efficacy of radical radiotherapy (conventional radiotherapy and SABR) plus 4 cycles of platinum-based doublet chemotherapy versus 4 cycles of platinum-based doublet chemotherapy alone in patients with oligometastatic NSCLC. Ablative radiotherapy will treat both the primary site and the oligometastatic site.

SUMMARY

In the absence of randomized data to guide appropriate management of oligometastatic NSCLC, patient selection for curative intent is primarily based on retrospective data derived from single-center experiences. The evidence thus far supports an aggressive curative posture for fit patients who present with a single organ site of synchronous (or metachronous) extrathoracic M1 disease and no evidence of intrathoracic lymph node involvement. Local control of both the primary and oligometastatic site can be achieved by either complete surgical resection or implementation of an ablative radiotherapy modality. A curative strategy for patients who harbor multiple synchronous or metachronous sites of oligometastatic NSCLC should be carefully considered on a case-by-case basis. Systemic chemotherapy is often used somewhere in this strategy, but the timing and efficacy remains unclear. Targeted chemotherapy (in addition to aggressive local control) should be strongly encouraged in the treatment strategy of patients with oligometastatic NSCLC who harbor sensitizing driver mutations. The key determinates of long-term survival include definitive treatment of the primary NSCLC, a single organ site of synchronous or metachronous disease, a long disease-free interval between treatment of the primary NSCLC and development of metastases, and the absence of intrathoracic lymph node (N0) disease.

Table 3 Location of oligometastases	
Location of Oligometastases	**N (%)**
Brain	269 (36)
Lung	254 (34)
Adrenal	98 (13)
Bone	64 (9)
Liver	18 (2)
Lymph node	18 (2)
Other	59 (8)

Data from Ashworth AB, Senan S, Palma DA, et al. An individual patient data meta-analysis of outcomes and prognostic factors after treatment of oligometastatic non-small-cell lung cancer. Clin Lung Cancer 2014;15(5):346–55.

REFERENCES

1. Carnio S, Novello S, Mele T, et al. Extending survival of stage IV non-small cell lung cancer. Semin Oncol 2014;41(1):69–92.
2. Morgensztern D, Campo MJ, Dahlberg SE, et al. Molecularly targeted therapies in non-small-cell lung cancer annual update 2014. J Thorac Oncol 2015;10(1 Suppl 1):S1–63.
3. Ashworth A, Rodrigues G, Boldt G, et al. Is there an oligometastatic state in non-small cell lung cancer? A systematic review of the literature. Lung Cancer 2013;82:197–203.
4. Hellman S, Weichselbaum RR. Oligometastases. J Clin Oncol 1995;13(1):8–10.
5. Macdermed DM, Weichselbaum RR, Salama JK. A rationale for the targeted treatment of oligometastases with radiotherapy. J Surg Oncol 2008;98:202–6.
6. Goldstraw P, Crowley J, Chansky K, et al. The IASLC lung cancer staging project: proposals for the revision of the TNM stage groupings in the forthcoming (seventh) edition of the TNM classification of malignant tumours. J Thorac Oncol 2007;2(8):706–14.
7. Eberhardt WE, Mitchell A, Crowley J, et al. The IASLC lung cancer staging project proposals for the revision of the m descriptors in the forthcoming eighth edition of the TNM classification of lung cancer. J Thorac Oncol 2015;10:1515–22.
8. Goldstraw P, Chansky K, Crowley J, et al. The IASLC lung cancer staging project: proposals for revision of the TNM stage groupings in the forthcoming (eighth) edition of the TNM classification for lung cancer. J Thorac Oncol 2016;11(1):39–51.
9. Tönnies M, Pfannschmidt J, Bauer TT, et al. Metastasectomy for synchronous solitary non-small cell lung cancer metastases. Ann Thorac Surg 2014; 98:249–56.
10. Congedo MT, Cesario A, Lococo F, et al. Surgery for oligometastatic NSCLC: long-term results from a single center experience. J Thorac Cardiovasc Surg 2012;144(2):444–52.
11. Downey RJ, Ng KK, Kris MG, et al. A phase II trial of chemotherapy and surgery for non-small cell lung cancer patients with a synchronous solitary metastasis. Lung Cancer 2002;38(2):193–7.
12. De Ruysscher D, Wanders R, van Baardwijk A, et al. Radical treatment of non-small-cell lung cancer patients with synchronous oligometastases: long-term results of a prospective phase II trial (Nct01282450). J Thorac Oncol 2012;7(10):1547–55.
13. Plönes T, Osei-Agyemang T, Krohn A, et al. Surgical treatment of extrapulmonary oligometastatic NSCLC. Indian J Surg 2015;77(Suppl 2):216–20.
14. Pericleous S, Mukhlerjee S, Hurchins RR. Lung adenocarcinoma presenting as obstructing jaundice: a case report and review of the literature. World J Surg Oncol 2008;6:120.
15. Mckeown PP, Conant P, Auerbach LE. Squamous cell carcinoma of the lung: an unusual metastasis to pectoralis muscle. Ann Thorac Surg 1996;61: 1525–6.
16. Luketich JD, Martini N, Ginsberg RJ, et al. Successful treatment of solitary extracranial metastases from NSCLC. Ann Thorac Surg 1995;60:1609–11.
17. Knights EM Jr. Metastatic tumors of the brain and their relation to primary and secondary pulmonary cancer. Cancer 1954;7:259.
18. Getman V, Devyatko E, Dunkler D, et al. Prognosis of patients with non-small cell lung cancer with isolated brain metastases undergoing combined surgical treatment. Eur J Cardiothorac Surg 2004;25:1107–13.
19. Billing PS, Miller DL, Allen MS, et al. Surgical treatment of primary lung cancer with synchronous brain metastases. J Thorac Cardiovasc Surg 2001;122: 548–53.
20. Bonnette P, Puyo P, Gabriel C, et al. Surgical management of non-small cell lung cancer with synchronous brain metastases. Chest 2001;119:1469–75.
21. Mussi A, Pistolesi M, Lucchi M, et al. Resection of single brain metastasis in non-small-cell lung cancer: prognostic factors. J Thorac Cardiovasc Surg 1996;112:146–53.
22. Burt M, Wronski M, Arbit E, et al. Resection of brain metastases from non-small-cell lung carcinoma: results of therapy. J Thorac Cardiovasc Surg 1992; 103:399–411.
23. Rossi NP, Zavala DC, VanGilder JC. A combined surgical approach to non-oat-cell pulmonary carcinoma with single cerebral metastasis. Respiration 1987;51:170–8.
24. Magilligan DJ Jr, Duvernoy C, Malik G, et al. Surgical approach to lung cancer with solitary cerebral metastasis: twenty-five years' experience. Ann Thorac Surg 1986;42:360–4.
25. Wroński M, Arbit E, Burt M, et al. Survival after surgical treatment of brain metastases from lung cancer: a follow-up study of 231 patients treated between 1976 and 1991. J Neurosurg 1995;83:605–16.
26. Patchell RA, Tibbs PA, Walsh JW, et al. A randomized trial of surgery in the treatment of single metastases to the brain. N Engl J Med 1990;322: 494–500.
27. Gaspar LE, Mehta MP, Patchell RA, et al. The role of whole brain radiation therapy in the management of newly diagnosed brain metastases: a systematic review and evidence-based clinical practice guideline. J Neurooncol 2010;96:17–32.
28. Linskey ME, Andrews DW, Asher AL, et al. The role of stereotactic radiosurgery in the management of patients with newly diagnosed brain metastases: a systematic review and evidence-based clinical practice guideline. J Neurooncol 2010;96:45–68 [Erratum appears in J Neurooncol 2010;96(1):69–70].

29. Kozower BD, Larner JM, Detterbeck FC, et al. Special treatment issues in NSCLC: diagnosis and management of lung cancer, 3rd ed. American College of Chest Physicians evidence-based clinical practice guidelines. Chest 2013;143(5 Suppl): e369S–99S.

30. Ettinger DS, Wood DE, Akerley W, et al. Non-small cell lung cancer, version 6.2015. J Natl Compr Canc Netw 2015;13(5):515–24.

31. Ettinghausen SE, Burt ME. Prospective evaluation of unilateral adrenal masses in patients with operable NSCLC. J Clin Oncol 1991;9(8):1462–6.

32. Singh PK, Buch HN. Adrenal incidentaloma: evaluation and management. J Clin Pathol 2008;61(11): 1168–73.

33. Kim HK, Choi YS, Kim K, et al. Preoperative evaluation of adrenal lesions based on imaging studies and laparoscopic adrenalectomy in patients with otherwise operable lung cancer. Lung Cancer 2007;58(3):342–7.

34. Pham DT, Dean DA, Detterbeck FC. Adrenalectomy as the new treatment paradigm for solitary adrenal metastasis from lung cancer. Paper presented at the 37th Annual Meeting of the Society of Thoracic Surgeons. New Orleans, LA, January 29–31, 2001.

35. Porte H, Siat J, Guibert B, et al. Resection of adrenal metastases from non-small cell lung cancer: a multicenter study. Ann Thorac Surg 2001;71(3):981–5.

36. Mercier O, Fadel E, de Perrot M, et al. Surgical treatment of solitary adrenal metastasis from non-small cell lung cancer. J Thorac Cardiovasc Surg 2005; 130(1):136–40.

37. Raz DJ, Lanuti M, Gaissert HC, et al. Outcomes of patients with isolated adrenal metastasis from non-small cell lung carcinoma. Ann Thorac Surg 2011; 92(5):1788–92.

38. Lucchi M, Dini P, Ambrogi MC, et al. Metachronous adrenal masses in resected non-small cell lung cancer patients: therapeutic implications of laparoscopic adrenalectomy. Eur J Cardiothorac Surg 2005;27(5): 753–6.

39. Howell GM, Carty SE, Armstrong MJ, et al. Outcome and prognostic factors after adrenalectomy for patients with distant adrenal metastasis. Ann Surg Oncol 2013;20(11):3491–6.

40. Strong VE, D'Angelica M, Tang L, et al. Laparoscopic adrenalectomy for isolated adrenal metastasis. Ann Surg Oncol 2007;14(12):3392–400.

41. Wade TP, Longo WE, Virgo KS, et al. A comparison of adrenalectomy with other resections for metastatic cancers. Am J Surg 1998;175(3):183–6.

42. Tanvetyanon T, Robinson LA, Schell MJ, et al. Outcomes of adrenalectomy for isolated synchronous versus metachronous adrenal metastases in non-small-cell lung cancer: a systematic review and pooled analysis. J Clin Oncol 2008;26(7): 1142–7.

43. Barone M, Di Nuzzo D, Cipollone G, et al. Oligometastatic non-small cell lung cancer (NSCLC): adrenal metastases. Experience in a single institution. Updates Surg 2015;67(4):383–7.

44. Meyer KK. Direct lymphatic connections from the lower lobes of the lung to the abdomen. J Thorac Surg 1958;35:726–33.

45. DeLuzio MR, Moores C, Dhamija A, et al. Resection of oligometastatic lung cancer to the pancreas may yield a survival benefit in select patients–a systematic review. Pancreatology 2015;15(5):456–62.

46. Ashworth AB, Senan S, Palma DA, et al. An individual patient data meta-analysis of outcomes and prognostic factors after treatment of oligometastatic non-small-cell lung cancer. Clin Lung Cancer 2014; 15(5):346–55.

47. Palma DA, Haasbeek CJ, Rodriques GB, et al. Stereotactic ablative radiotherapy for comprehensive treatment of oligometastatic tumors (SABR-COMET): study protocol for a randomized phase II trial. BMC Cancer 2012;12:305.

The Role of Induction Therapy for Esophageal Cancer

Mark F. Berry, MD

KEYWORDS

- Esophageal neoplasms • Induction therapy • Esophagectomy

KEY POINTS

- Induction therapy before esophagectomy has been extensively investigated and increasingly used, and may be partially responsible for the recent improvements noted for the prognosis of esophageal cancer.
- Induction therapy does not seem to have a role for superficial cancers without lymph node involvement, but several randomized trials found a benefit for more locally advanced but resectable tumors.
- Induction chemoradiation is recommended before esophagectomy for locally advanced squamous cell carcinoma.
- Both induction chemotherapy and induction chemoradiation are found to be beneficial for locally advanced adenocarcinoma. Neither strategy has a clear advantage, but consensus-based guidelines currently recommend induction chemoradiation for this clinical scenario.

INTRODUCTION

The incidence of esophageal cancer is increasing, with an estimated 16,980 new cases in the United States in 2012.[1–4] Esophageal cancer staging is currently defined by the most recent seventh edition American Joint Committee on Cancer (AJCC) TNM Staging System (**Table 1**), which classifies Barret's esophagus with high-grade dysplasia as T_{is} and also stages esophagogastric junction (EGJ) tumors, defined as those tumors arising at the EGJ or in the cardia of the stomach within 5 cm of the EGJ that extend into the EGJ or esophagus, as esophageal cancers.[5] Surgery with esophagectomy is considered the standard of care for localized disease and is the best single-modality therapy for potentially resectable disease. Overall 5-year survival for patients with esophageal cancer is generally poor, although improvement has been observed over time with an increase from 5% to 17% to 19% over the last 4 decades.[2–4] These survival improvements have likely partly resulted from earlier detection in the setting of Barrett's esophagus and improvements in perioperative care. However, the recently improved prognosis is also likely partially caused by the demonstration of the benefits and the subsequent use of multimodality therapy for specific stages of esophageal cancer.

The poor survival rate after esophagectomy alone for patients with locally advanced but not metastatic disease led to many studies of multimodality therapy in efforts to improve outcomes.[6] The use of chemotherapy and radiation therapy has been investigated in the preoperative and postoperative settings. Adjuvant therapies, with either chemotherapy or radiotherapy, have not shown survival benefits.[7] However, induction therapy used before esophagectomy has been

There are no disclosures or potential conflicts to report.
Department of Cardiothoracic Surgery, Stanford University, 870 Quarry Road, Falk Cardiovascular Research Building, 2nd Floor, Stanford, CA 94305, USA
E-mail address: berry037@stanford.edu

Thorac Surg Clin 26 (2016) 295–304
http://dx.doi.org/10.1016/j.thorsurg.2016.04.006

Table 1
T, N, and M status and histologic grade definitions for esophagus and esophagogastric junction cancer in the seventh edition of the AJCC Cancer Staging Manual

T Status	
T_{is}	High-grade dysplasia
T1	Invasion into the lamina propria, muscularis mucosae, or submucosa
T2	Invasion into muscularis propria
T3	Invasion into adventitia
T4a	Invades resectable adjacent structures (pleura, pericardium, diaphragm)
T4b	Invades unresectable adjacent structures (aorta, vertebral body, trachea)
N status	
N0	No regional lymph node metastases
N1	1–2 positive regional lymph nodes
N2	3–6 positive regional lymph nodes
N3	7 or more positive regional lymph nodes
M status	
M0	No distant metastases
M1	Distant metastases
Histologic grade	
G1	Well differentiated
G2	Moderately differentiated
G3	Poorly differentiated
G4	Undifferentiated

hypothesized to potentially downstage and control local and micrometastatic disease and, therefore, be more beneficial than adjuvant therapy. This hypothesis is partly supported by the belief that chemotherapy and radiation are better tolerated before rather than after esophagectomy. In addition, the use of induction therapy may allow potentially morbid surgery to be avoided in patients with unfavorable biology who show progression of disease through induction therapy.

Many studies have investigated the use of induction therapy before esophagectomy for esophageal cancer. Not all of these studies found a benefit to induction therapy, but several did, and induction therapy is currently used in most patients who have locally advanced esophageal cancer.[8] This article reviews the evidence and guidelines related to the use of either chemotherapy or radiation therapy before esophagectomy for esophageal cancer.

ROLE OF INDUCTION THERAPY

Surgery is considered integral to achieving cure in patients with esophageal cancer.[9–11] Randomized trials comparing surgical versus nonsurgical treatment have not been performed, but a study from the linked Surveillance, Epidemiology, and End-Results (SEER)-Medicare database found that 5-year survival rates for patients with stages I through III esophageal cancer treated with and without surgery were 28% and 10%, respectively.[10] Although these data may reflect a selection bias in which surgically treated patients had better survival because they were younger and healthier, definitive chemoradiation is generally reserved for those patients who refuse surgery or are not surgical candidates.[12] The only area of esophageal cancer in which definitive chemoradiation is recommended in place of surgical resection is squamous cell carcinoma of the cervical esophagus.[12,13] Some data suggest that definitive chemoradiation could be adequate for some patients with squamous cell carcinoma in other esophageal locations, but surgery is considered integral to potential cure for adenocarcinoma in which pathologic complete response rates are generally less common.[14–16]

However long-term outcomes are generally not considered satisfactory with resection alone, even if microscopically complete (R0), except for early-stage superficial cancers without lymph node involvement.[17] These poor outcomes have fueled many investigations into the use of induction therapy to try and improve survival. As will be discussed in detail later, many studies failed to show a definitive benefit to induction therapy, and the level of evidence supporting the use of induction therapy remains somewhat limited. Despite the limited evidence, the use of induction therapy has been supported by meta-analyses and remained an active area in research, with additional trials being performed, and in clinical practice.[18,19] The use of induction chemoradiation in the United States steadily increased from 2003 to 2011, which was a period in which published studies supporting the practice were generally limited in number.[8]

A complicating feature of establishing the optimal treatment for esophageal cancer is the heterogeneous nature of this disease. Squamous cell carcinoma was historically the most common histology seen with a location somewhat evenly distributed throughout the distal two-thirds of the esophagus. Epidemiologic shifts in the last few decades have led to adenocarcinomas of the distal esophagus or EGJ to be the most common clinical entity of esophageal cancer seen in the United States.[20] Patients with adenocarcinoma and squamous cell carcinoma were observed to have similar long-term survival across major treatment modalities, and treatment guidelines for adenocarcinoma and squamous cell carcinoma were, therefore, previously essentially equivalent.[21]

However, clinical subsets of histology and tumor location are increasingly recognized as likely separate disease entities within the spectrum of esophageal cancer. The optimal therapy for esophageal cancer, including not only specific surgical technique but also specific radiation therapy or systemic therapy, may vary according to stage and specific histology and tumor location. For example, the optimal treatment of adenocarcinoma at the distal esophagus or the EGJ possibly related to obesity or reflux is probably different than that for a proximal or midesophageal squamous cell carcinoma possibly related to tobacco or alcohol use. The 2 histologic subtypes now have separate stage groupings and treatment algorithms in the latest, revised staging system and in the National Comprehensive Cancer Network (NCCN) treatment guidelines (**Table 2**).[5,12,22] However, the rarity of esophageal cancer has led most trials for practical enrollment purposes to have a wide inclusion criteria in terms of histology and tumor location.[23–25] The inclusion of heterogeneous clinical entities in most clinical trials not only impacts the generalizability of the trial results but may also have prevented the trials from demonstrating benefits that could be used to define optimal multimodality therapy.

Another complicating feature of establishing the optimal treatment of esophageal cancer is the heterogeneity of available therapies. Esophageal resection can be performed via several different techniques, with the most appropriate technique for any specific patient being dependent on both patient and surgeon factors. There are also many induction therapy options with regard to chemotherapeutic agents, radiation dose and other treatment details, and whether radiation is combined with chemotherapy and, if so, the timing. Most studies have some variation in the use of chemotherapy or radiation therapy, which creates some difficulties when trying to compare the studies' findings or derive definitive conclusions from the pooled results of the studies. Most studies have also compared induction therapy of some kind with surgery alone, and few studies have compared induction chemotherapy with induction chemoradiation. Perhaps the only opinion of induction therapy that is universally accepted is that induction radiation alone is not recommended, based on studies that evaluated radiation alone as induction therapy or compared radiation alone and chemoradiation either as definitive management or as an induction therapy.[12,26–28]

Table 2
AJCC seventh edition stage groupings

	Adenocarcinoma				Squamous Cell Carcinoma				
Stage	T	N	M	Grade	T	N	M	G	Location
0	is	0	0	1	is	0	0	1	Any
IA	1	0	0	1–2	1	0	0	1	Any
IB	1	0	0	3	1	0	0	2–3	Any
	2	0	0	1–2	2–3	0	0	1	Lower
IIA	2	0	0	3	2–3	0	0	1	Upper Middle
	—	—	—	—	2–3	0	0	2–3	Lower
IIB	3	0	0	Any	2–3	0	0	2–3	Upper Middle
	1–2	1	0	Any	1–2	1	0	Any	Any
IIIA	1–2	2	0	Any	1–2	2	0	Any	Any
	3	1	0	Any	3	1	0	Any	Any
	4a	0	0	Any	4a	0	0	Any	Any
IIIB	3	2	0	Any	3	2	0	Any	Any
IIIC	4a	1–2	0	Any	4a	1–2	0	Any	Any
	4b	Any	0	Any	4b	Any	0	Any	Any
	Any	3	0	Any	Any	3	0	Any	Any
IV	Any	Any	1	Any	Any	Any	1	Any	Any

Cancer location definitions: Upper thoracic, 20 to 25 cm from incisors; middle thoracic, 25 to 30 cm from incisors; lower thoracic, 30 to 40 cm from incisors.

Induction Chemotherapy

Several trials investigated the use of induction chemotherapy for esophageal cancer—8 of these trials are listed in **Table 3**.[23,29–35] Four of these 8 trials showed a benefit to induction chemotherapy. The trials varied in terms of both specific agents and number of cycles, and the trials also varied by the histology and tumor location included in the study. The actual treatment received within each specific trial was also not uniform; for example, only approximately 50% of patients enrolled on the Medical Research Council Adjuvant Gastric Infusional Chemotherapy (MAGIC) trial received all 3 planned postoperative chemotherapy courses.[23]

As shown in **Table 3**, 3 randomized trials have investigated the use of induction chemotherapy for esophageal squamous cell carcinoma. Two of these studies did not find a benefit.[29,30] The third study did show that patients treated with induction therapy had improved 5-year survival rates compared with patients treated with surgery (26% vs 17%; $P = .03$).[31] Despite the positive finding, interestingly, the study was conducted from 1989 to 1996 but did not have the final results published until 2011 because of changes in study personnel and loss of interest in the chemotherapy regimen.[31] As also shown in **Table 3**, 2 large randomized trials (the Medical Research Council OE2 trial of surgery with or without preoperative chemotherapy for esophageal cancer and the North American RTOG 8911/Intergroup 113 trial) investigated the use of induction chemotherapy in a mixed cohort of adenocarcinoma and squamous cell carcinoma.[9,32,33,36] The Intergroup study found no benefit, and the other study found a modest benefit (23% vs 17% 5-year survival rates; $P = .004$).

Several randomized trials evaluated the use of induction chemotherapy for adenocarcinoma of the distal esophagus or the EGJ (see **Table 3**).[23,34,35] Interpreting the impact of induction therapy for esophageal cancer must be done somewhat cautiously, as these studies were either designed primarily for or included a significant number of patients with gastric cancer. The epidemiologic and biologic differences between distal esophageal/EGJ and noncardia gastric adenocarcinomas may preclude the extrapolation of results from predominantly gastric cancer trials to distal esophageal or EGJ tumors.[37] Of these 3 trials of perioperative chemotherapy versus surgery alone in patients with gastric cancer that included individuals with distal esophageal or EGJ tumors, 2 showed a survival benefit for this approach (the MAGIC and French Federation Nationale des Centres de Lutte Centre le Cancer/Federation Francophone de Cancerologie

---

Table 3
Randomized trials of induction chemotherapy that included esophageal cancer patients

Author, Year	Patients	Histology	Induction Therapy	Survival Benefit
SCC patients only				
Law et al,[29] 1997	74 IT 73 surgery	SCC	Cis/5-FU	None (17 vs 13 mo MS)
Ancona et al,[30] 2001	48 IT 48 surgery	SCC	Cis/5-FU	None
Boonstra et al,[31] 2011	85 IT 84 surgery	SCC	Cis/Etop	26% vs 17% 5-y survival
SCC and AC patients				
Kelsen et al,[32] 1998	216 IT 227 surgery	SCC & AC	Cis/5-FU	None (MS 1.3 y in both groups)
Allum et al,[33] 2009	400 IT 402 surgery	SCC & AC	Cis/5-FU	23% vs 17% 5-y survival
AC patients only (also included gastric adenocarcinoma)				
Cunningham et al,[23] 2006	250 IT 253 surgery	AC (26% EGJ/ esophageal)	ECF	36% vs 23% 5-y survival
Ychou et al,[34] 2011	113 IT 111 surgery	AC (75% EGJ/ esophageal)	Cis/5-FU	38% vs 24% 5-y survival
Schuhmacher et al,[35] 2010	72 IT 72 surgery	AC (53% EGJ)	Cis/5-FU	None

Abbreviations: 5-FU, fluorouracil; AC, adenocarcinoma; cis, cisplatin; ECF, epirubicin/cisplatin/5-FU; Etop, Etoposide; IT, induction therapy; MS, median survival; SCC, squamous cell carcinoma.

Digestive [FNLCC/FFCD] trials[23,34]), while a third (European Organisation for Research and Treatment of Cancer [EORTC] trial 40,954) did not.[35]

The European MAGIC trial showed the survival benefit of perioperative chemotherapy with epirubicin, cisplatin, and fluorouracil in patients with distal esophageal, EGJ, and gastric adenocarcinoma.[23] The success of this trial raised questions as to whether radiotherapy was a necessary component of gastric and EGJ cancer treatment, although 74% of patients in the trial had gastric cancers. This trial required postoperative chemotherapy, but only 42% of surgical patients were able to complete the planned 3 cycles of the postoperative chemotherapy. Patients treated with perioperative chemotherapy had a 25% reduction in the risk of death that translated into an improvement in 5-year survival from 23% to 36%. A similar benefit for neoadjuvant chemotherapy was noted in a French multicenter FNLCC/FFCD trial in which 224 patients with potentially resectable stage II or greater adenocarcinoma of the stomach (n = 55), EGJ (n = 144), or distal esophagus (n = 25) were randomly assigned to 2 to 3 cycles of preoperative chemotherapy or surgery alone.[34] At a median 5.7-year follow-up, neoadjuvant chemotherapy was associated with a significant 35% reduction in the risk of disease recurrence, and 5-year survival

rate was also significantly better in the chemotherapy group (38% vs 24%).

A third trial that investigated the use of induction chemotherapy for gastric adenocarcinoma but included EGJ patients closed prematurely because of poor accrual and did not find a survival difference between study groups.[35] However, a survival benefit for neoadjuvant chemotherapy was shown in a 2011 meta-analysis that included 9 randomized comparisons of neoadjuvant chemotherapy versus surgery alone for esophageal or EGJ cancers.[19] The hazard ratio for all-cause mortality for neoadjuvant chemotherapy was 0.87 (95% confidence interval, 0.70–0.88), and this translated into an absolute survival benefit at 2 years of 5.1%. These data support a significant survival benefit for neoadjuvant chemotherapy over surgery alone.

Induction Chemoradiation

Trials have also investigated the use of induction chemotherapy combined with radiation therapy for esophageal cancer. Combining radiation with induction chemotherapy has the potential benefit of improving local control and being more likely to obtain a complete pathologic response while still providing systemic control. Ten of these trials are listed in **Table 4**.[24,25,38–45] As shown in the

Table 4
Selected randomized trials of induction chemoradiation therapy for esophageal cancer

Author, Year	Patients	Histology	Induction Chemotherapy	Induction RT	Survival Benefit
Nygaard et al,[38] 1992	41 IT 47 surgery	SCC	Cis/bleo	35 Gy	None (17% vs 9% 3-y survival)
Le Prise et al,[39] 1994	45 IT 41 surgery	SCC	Cis/5-FU	20 Gy	None (19% vs 14% 3-y survival)
Apinop et al,[40] 1994	34 IT 35 surgery	SCC	Cis/5-FU	40 Gy	None (26% vs 20% 3-y survival)
Bosset et al,[41] 1997	139 IT 143 surgery	SCC	Cis	37 Gy	None (36% vs 34% 3-y survival)
Walsh et al,[42] 1996	55 IT 58 surgery	AC	Cis/5-FU	40 Gy	32% vs 6% 3-y survival
Urba et al,[43] 2001	50 IT 50 surgery	SCC & AC	Cis/5-FU/vinbl	45 Gy	None (30% vs 16% 3-year survival)
Burmeister et al,[25] 2005	128 IT 128 surgery	SCC & AC	Cis/5-FU	35 Gy	None (22 vs 19 mo MS)
Tepper et al,[44] 2008	30 IT 26 surgery	SCC & AC	Cis/5-FU	50.4 Gy	39% vs 16% 5-y survival
Van Hagen et al,[24] 2012	178 IT 188 surgery	SCC & AC	Cis/Pac	41.4 Gy	49 vs 24 mo MS
Mariette et al,[45] 2014	98 IT 97 surgery	SCC & AC	Cis/5-FU	45 Gy	None (48 vs 53% 3-y survival)

Abbreviations: 5-FU, fluorouracil; AC, adenocarcinoma; bleo, bleomycin; cis, cisplatin; IT, induction therapy; pac, paclitaxel; RT, radiotherapy; SCC, squamous cell carcinoma; vinbl, vinblastine.

table, the trials varied by the specific induction therapy used and which histologies and tumor locations were included.

Four trials of induction chemoradiation for esophageal squamous cell carcinoma were published in the 1990s, with none of the trials finding a benefit to induction chemoradiation.[38–41] It is hypothesized that some of the reasons for failing to find a benefit to induction chemoradiation in these earlier studies are suboptimal staging modalities that understaged patients, nonstandardization of surgical approaches, and induction treatment regimens that are now considered outdated.[45] It wasn't until 1996 that a positive trial was reported.[42] In this trial, 58 patients with adenocarcinoma of the esophagus were randomly assigned to surgery alone or multimodality therapy, with multimodality patients having better 3-year survival rates (32% vs 6%). Despite the positive findings, one concern regarding this trial was that the benefits of induction chemotherapy were potentially overestimated by the somewhat unexpected poor survival observed in the patients treated with surgery alone. Another trial around the same time found what seemed to be a clinically substantial benefit to induction chemoradiation (30% vs 16% 3-year survival rates), but the difference was not statistically significant, and the study was considered to have likely been underpowered.[43]

Trial CALGB 9781 had poor accrual and was closed prematurely but ultimately found that 5-year survival was better with trimodality therapy compared with surgery alone (39% vs 16%).[44] However, the largest and most influential trial supporting the use of induction chemoradiation for esophageal cancer is the Dutch Chemoradiotherapy for Oesophageal Cancer followed by Surgery Study (CROSS) trial.[24] This trial randomly assigned 363 patients (24% squamous cell carcinoma, 75% adenocarcinoma) with potentially resectable distal esophageal (89%) or EGJ cancer (11%) to preoperative chemoradiation versus surgery alone. The complete (R0) resection rate was higher with chemoradiation (92% vs 65%). The study's results were first reported at a median follow-up of 32 months, at which time overall survival was found to be significantly better with preoperative chemoradiation (3-year survival rate, 58% vs 44%). The survival benefit persisted with longer (median, 84-month) follow-up (5-year survival rate, 47% vs 33%).[46]

In contrast, other large trials have not shown a significant survival advantage for the neoadjuvant chemoradiation approach compared with surgery alone.[25,45] One of these trials, FFCD 9901, was a multicenter, randomized trial of 195 patients who were treated with surgery alone and 98 patients treated with 45 Gy of radiation and 2 courses of concomitant chemotherapy followed by surgery.[45] The trial was stopped earlier than planned for anticipated futility when interim analysis found an improbability of demonstrating superiority of either treatment arm with regard to the primary endpoint of overall survival, and ultimately no difference in 3-year overall survival was seen between the 2 treatment arms (3-year overall survival rate, 53% vs 47.5%; $P = .94$). This trial was limited to patients with stage I or II disease according to the fifth staging edition definitions. Patients in this trial treated with induction therapy had a higher postoperative mortality rate than the patients treated with surgery alone (11.1% vs 3.4%; $P = .049$). However, overall, several meta-analyses support a survival benefit for neoadjuvant concurrent chemoradiation compared with surgery alone for esophageal and EGJ cancer.[19,47] One meta-analysis estimates an absolute survival benefit of 8.7% at 2 years for neoadjuvant chemoradiation.[19] Survival benefit to induction chemoradiation was also found in a retrospective National Cancer Database study (5-year survival rate, 37.9% vs 28.7%).[8]

Induction Chemotherapy Versus Induction Chemoradiation

As discussed above, there is some evidence that both induction chemotherapy and induction chemoradiation have benefit before esophagectomy for esophageal cancer. Very few studies have been conducted to directly compare the 2 induction strategies. The German POET trial randomly assigned patients with T3-4NXM0 adenocarcinoma of the lower esophagus, EGJ, or gastric cardia to neoadjuvant chemotherapy with cisplatin, fluorouracil, and leucovorin or neoadjuvant chemoradiation (12 weeks of the cisplatin/fluorouracil/leucovorin regimen and then 3 weeks of 30-Gy radiation concurrent with cisplatin/etoposide).[48] The study closed prematurely because of poor accrual and found an improvement in survival for chemoradiation that was not statistically significant (3-year survival rate, 47% vs 28%; $P = .07$). Another trial that addressed the relative benefits of preoperative chemotherapy versus chemoradiation was a randomized phase II Australian trial involving 75 patients with adenocarcinoma of the esophagus or EGJ in which no significant difference in median overall survival was found (32 vs 29 months).[49] A meta-analysis of these 2 trials did not find a statistically significant difference in survival between the 2 regimens.[19] Another randomized trial is currently being conducted in Europe, Canada, and Australia to directly compare preoperative chemotherapy alone versus chemoradiation in patients with resectable adenocarcinoma of the stomach and EGJ.[50] For now, the relative benefits of preoperative chemotherapy versus chemoradiation for esophageal adenocarcinoma remain uncertain.

Another area of active research is the use of targeted therapy in the induction setting. The addition of trastuzumab to first-line chemotherapy for patients with advanced nonsurgical gastric or EGJ cancer whose tumors had overexpression of the HER2 protein is found to provide a modest but statistically significant survival benefit over chemotherapy alone (13.8 vs 11.1 months; $P = .0046$).[51] The TRAP study is a feasibility study currently being conducted to evaluate the addition of the targeted agents trastuzumab and pertuzumab to standard induction chemoradiation for HER2+ resectable esophageal cancer.[52]

SELECTING THERAPY

The prognosis for patients treated for intra- and submucosal (T1) esophageal cancers is significantly better than the prognosis for all other patients found to have esophageal cancer, even those also found in other relatively early-stage disease.[5] Patients with these superficial esophageal cancers are typically recommended to undergo endoscopic resection if possible or surgery without induction treatment.[12] This strategy is supported both by the excellent outcomes seen with local therapy alone[17] and the fact that multimodality trials that focused/included earlier stage patients did not show a benefit to induction therapy.[39,41,45]

The use of induction therapy for clinical T2N0 (cT2N0) tumors has been increasing but is somewhat controversial, as both clinical understaging and clinical overstaging are common in these patients.[22,53–59] The CROSS trial that showed benefit to induction chemoradiation did include cT2N0 patients, although they were only 17% of enrolled patients.[24] However, several studies that restricted analysis to cT2N0 patients found no survival benefit to induction therapy over surgery alone.[59,60] Consistent with the uncertainty of optimal treatment, the NCCN guidelines for medically fit patients allow a wide spectrum of treatment possibilities that include definitive chemoradiation and esophagectomy with or without induction or adjuvant therapy.[12] However, many clinicians use a strategy of surgery for these patients and consideration of adjuvant therapy for patients who are upstaged or otherwise thought to be at high risk for metastatic disease.[53]

However, patients with T1-2N0M0 tumors are a minority of patients who present with potentially resectable disease.[5,20] Most patients who do not have metastatic disease have what is considered to be locoregional or locally advanced disease (T3-4aN0, T1-4aN1M0). The NCCN guidelines reflect a lack of available definitive data on the optimal treatment and essentially consider any combination of esophagectomy and chemoradiation or even definitive chemoradiation as acceptable therapy.[12] Not surprisingly, the treatment of these patients is highly variable in practice.[61] However, as described above, evidence that induction therapy followed by surgical resection is the optimal treatment of patients with T3-4a tumors or nodal disease is accumulating. Currently, induction chemoradiation is recommended for squamous cell carcinoma patients with this extent of disease.[12] Induction therapy is also recommended for patients with locally advanced adenocarcinoma. Although a clear advantage of chemoradiation over chemotherapy alone has not been found, consensus-based NCCN guidelines derived from the evidence listed above state a preference for preoperative chemoradiation over preoperative chemotherapy alone for patients with esophageal or EGJ adenocarcinoma and this extent of disease.

SUMMARY

Survival of esophageal cancer generally is poor but has been improving. Induction therapy before esophagectomy has been extensively investigated and increasingly used and may be partially responsible for the recently observed improved prognosis. Induction therapy does not seem to have a role for superficial cancers without lymph node involvement, but the results of several randomized trials support its use for more locally advanced tumors that are resectable. Induction chemoradiation is recommended before esophagectomy for locally advanced squamous cell carcinoma. Both induction chemotherapy and induction chemoradiation are found to be beneficial for locally advanced adenocarcinoma. Although a clear advantage of either strategy has not yet been found, consensus-based guidelines currently recommend induction chemoradiation for locally advanced adenocarcinoma.

REFERENCES

1. Siegel RL, Miller KD, Jemal A. Cancer statistics, 2015. CA Cancer J Clin 2015;65:5–29.
2. Howlader N, Noone AM, Krapcho M, et al. SEER cancer statistics review 1975-2013, National Cancer Institute, Bethesda, MD, http:/seer.cancer.gov/csr/1975-2013/, based on November 2015 SEER data submission, posted to the SEER website, April 2016.

3. Dubecz A, Gall I, Solymosi N, et al. Temporal trends in long-term survival and cure rates in esophageal cancer: a SEER database analysis. J Thorac Oncol 2012;7:443–7.

4. Pennathur A, Luketich JD. Resection for esophageal cancer: strategies for optimal management. Ann Thorac Surg 2008;85:S751–6.

5. Rice TW, Rusch VW, Ishwaran H, et al. Cancer of the esophagus and esophagogastric junction: data-driven staging for the seventh edition of the American Joint Committee on Cancer/International Union Against Cancer Cancer Staging Manuals. Cancer 2010;116:3763–73.

6. Kleinberg L, Forastiere AA. Chemoradiation in the management of esophageal cancer. Clin Oncol 2007;25:4110–7.

7. Mariette C, Piessen G, Triboulet JP. Therapeutic strategies in oesophageal carcinoma: Role of surgery and other modalities. Lancet Oncol 2007;8:545–53.

8. Speicher PJ, Wang X, Englum BR, et al. Induction chemoradiation therapy prior to esophagectomy is associated with superior long-term survival for esophageal cancer. Dis Esophagus 2014;28(8):788–96.

9. Kelsen DP, Winter KA, Gunderson LL, et al. Long-term results of RTOG trial 8911 (USA Intergroup 113): a random assignment trial comparison of chemotherapy followed by surgery compared with surgery alone for esophageal cancer. J Clin Oncol 2007;25:3719–25.

10. Paulson EC, Ra J, Armstrong K, et al. Underuse of esophagectomy as treatment for resectable esophageal cancer. Arch Surg 2008;143:1198–203.

11. Abrams JA, Buono DL, Strauss J, et al. Esophagectomy compared with chemoradiation for early stage esophageal cancer in the elderly. Cancer 2009;115:4924–33.

12. Ajani JA, D'Amico TA, Almhanna K, et al. Esophageal and esophagogastric junction cancers. J Natl Compr Canc Netw 2015;13:194–227.

13. Tong DKH, Law S, Kwong DLW, et al. Current management of cervical esophageal cancer. World J Surg 2011;35:600–7.

14. Bedenne L, Michel P, Bouche O, et al. Chemoradiation followed by surgery compared with chemoradiation alone in squamous cancer of the esophagus: FFCD 9102. J Clin Oncol 2007;25:1160–8.

15. Stahl M, Stuschke M, Lehmann N, et al. Chemoradiation with and without surgery in patients with locally advanced squamous cell carcinoma of the esophagus. J Clin Oncol 2005;23:2310–7.

16. Castoro C, Scarpa M, Cagol M, et al. Complete clinical response after neoadjuvant chemoradiotherapy for squamous cell cancer of the thoracic oesophagus: is surgery always necessary? J Gastrointest Surg 2013;17:1375–81.

17. Berry MF, Zeyer-Brunner J, Castleberry AW, et al. Treatment modalities for T1N0 esophageal cancers: a comparative analysis of local therapy versus surgical resection. J Thorac Oncol 2013;8:796–802.

18. Iyer R, Wilkinson N, Demmy T, et al. Controversies in the multimodality management of locally advanced esophageal cancer: evidence-based review of surgery alone and combined-modality therapy. Ann Surg Oncol 2004;11:665–73.

19. Sjoquist KM, Burmeister BH, Smithers BM, et al. Survival after neoadjuvant chemotherapy or chemoradiotherapy for resectable oesophageal carcinoma: an updated meta-analysis. Lancet Oncol 2011;12:681–92.

20. Enzinger PC, Mayer RJ. Esophageal cancer. N Engl J Med 2003;349:2241–52.

21. Chang DT, Chapman C, Shen J, et al. Treatment of esophageal cancer based on histology: a surveillance epidemiology and end results analysis. Am J Clin Oncol 2009;32:405–10.

22. Berry MF. Esophageal cancer: staging system and guidelines for staging and treatment. J Thorac Dis 2014;6(Suppl 3):S289–97.

23. Cunningham D, Allum WH, Stenning SP, et al. Perioperative chemotherapy versus surgery alone for resectable gastroesophageal cancer. N Engl J Med 2006;355:11.

24. van Hagen P, Hulshof MC, van Lanschot JJ, et al. Preoperative chemoradiotherapy for esophageal or junctional cancer. N Engl J Med 2012;366:2074–84.

25. Burmeister BH, Smithers BM, Gebski V, et al. Surgery alone versus chemoradiotherapy followed by surgery for resectable cancer of the oesophagus: a randomised controlled phase III trial. Lancet Oncol 2005;6:659–68.

26. Cooper JS, Guo MD, Herskovic A, et al. Chemoradiotherapy of locally advanced esophageal cancer: long-term follow-up of a prospective randomized trial (RTOG 85-01). Radiation Therapy Oncology Group. JAMA 1999;281:1623–7.

27. Herskovic A, Martz K, al-Sarraf M, et al. Combined chemotherapy and radiotherapy compared with radiotherapy alone in patients with cancer of the esophagus. N Engl J Med 1992;326:1593–8.

28. Arnott SJ, Duncan W, Gignoux M, et al. Preoperative radiotherapy for esophageal carcinoma. Cochrane Database Syst Rev 2005;(4):CD001799.

29. Law S, Fok M, Chow S, et al. Preoperative chemotherapy versus surgical therapy alone for squamous cell carcinoma of the esophagus: a prospective randomized trial. J Thorac Cardiovasc Surg 1997;114:210–7.

30. Ancona E, Ruol A, Santi S, et al. Only pathologic complete response to neoadjuvant chemotherapy improves significantly the long term survival of patients with resectable esophageal squamous cell carcinoma: final report of a randomized, controlled

trial of preoperative chemotherapy versus surgery alone. Cancer 2001;91:2165–74.

31. Boonstra JJ, Kok TC, Wijnhoven BP, et al. Chemotherapy followed by surgery versus surgery alone in patients with resectable oesophageal squamous cell carcinoma: long-term results of a randomized controlled trial. BMC Cancer 2011;11:181.

32. Kelsen DP, Ginsberg R, Pajak TF, et al. Chemotherapy followed by surgery compared with surgery alone for localized esophageal cancer. N Engl J Med 1998;339:1979.

33. Allum WH, Stenning SP, Bancewicz J, et al. Long-term results of a randomized trial of surgery with or without preoperative chemotherapy in esophageal cancer. J Clin Oncol 2009;27:5062.

34. Ychou M, Boige V, Pignon JP, et al. Perioperative chemotherapy compared with surgery alone for resectable gastroesophageal adenocarcinoma: an FNCLCC and FFCD multicenter phase III trial. J Clin Oncol 2011;29:1715.

35. Schuhmacher C, Gretschel S, Lordick F, et al. Neoadjuvant chemotherapy compared with surgery alone for locally advanced cancer of the stomach and cardia: European Organisation for Research and Treatment of Cancer randomized trial 40954. J Clin Oncol 2010;28:5210.

36. Medical Research Council Oesophageal Cancer Working Group. Surgical resection with or without preoperative chemotherapy in oesophageal cancer: a randomised controlled trial. Lancet 2002; 359:1727.

37. Whiteman DC, Parmar P, Fahey P, et al. Association of Helicobacter pylori infection with reduced risk for esophageal cancer is independent of environmental and genetic modifiers. Gastroenterology 2010;139:73.

38. Nygaard K, Hagen S, Hansen HS, et al. Pre-operative radiotherapy prolongs survival in operable esophageal carcinoma: a randomized, multicenter study of pre-operative radiotherapy and chemotherapy. The second Scandinavian trial in esophageal cancer. World J Surg 1992;16:1104–9.

39. Le Prise E, Etienne PL, Meunier B, et al. A randomized study of chemotherapy, radiation therapy, and surgery versus surgery for localized squamous cell carcinoma of the esophagus. Cancer 1994;73:1779–84.

40. Apinop C, Puttisak P, Preecha N. A prospective study of combined therapy in esophageal cancer. Hepatogastroenterology 1994;41:391–3.

41. Bosset JF, Gignoux M, Triboulet JP, et al. Chemoradiotherapy followed by surgery compared with surgery alone in squamous-cell cancer of the esophagus. N Engl J Med 1997;337:161–7.

42. Walsh TN, Noonan N, Hollywood D, et al. A comparison of multimodal therapy and surgery for esophageal adenocarcinoma. N Engl J Med 1996;335:462–7.

43. Urba SG, Orringer MB, Turrisi A, et al. Randomized trial of preoperative chemoradiation versus surgery alone in patients with locoregional esophageal carcinoma. J Clin Oncol 2001;19:305.

44. Tepper J, Krasna MJ, Niedzwiecki D, et al. Phase III trial of trimodality therapy with cisplatin, fluorouracil, radiotherapy, and surgery compared with surgery alone for esophageal cancer: CALGB 9781. J Clin Oncol 2008;26:1086–92.

45. Mariette C, Dahan L, Mornex F, et al. Surgery alone versus chemoradiotherapy followed by surgery for stage I and II esophageal cancer: final analysis of randomized controlled phase III trial FFCD 9901. J Clin Oncol 2014;32:2416–22.

46. Shapiro J, van Lanschot JJ, Hulshof MC, et al. Neoadjuvant chemoradiotherapy plus surgery versus surgery alone for oesophageal or junctional cancer (CROSS): long-term results of a randomised controlled trial. Lancet Oncol 2015; 16:1090.

47. Ronellenfitsch U, Schwarzbach M, Hofheinz R, et al. Perioperative chemo(radio)therapy versus primary surgery for resectable adenocarcinoma of the stomach, gastroesophageal junction, and lower esophagus. Cochrane Database Syst Rev 2013;5: CD008107.

48. Stahl M, Walz MK, Stuschke M, et al. Phase III comparison of preoperative chemotherapy compared with chemoradiotherapy in patients with locally advanced adenocarcinoma of the esophagogastric junction. J Clin Oncol 2009;27:851.

49. Burmeister BH, Thomas JM, Burmeister EA, et al. Is concurrent radiation therapy required in patients receiving preoperative chemotherapy for adenocarcinoma of the oesophagus? A randomised phase II trial. Eur J Cancer 2011;47:354.

50. Leong T, Smithers M, Michael M, et al. TOPGEAR: an international randomized phase III trial of preoperative chemoradiotherapy versus preoperative chemotherapy flor resectable gastric cancer (AGITG/TROG/EORTC/NCIC CTG). J Clin Oncol 2012;30(Suppl):TPS4141.

51. Bang YJ, Van Cutsem E, Feyereislova A, et al. Trastuzumab in combination with chemotherapy versus chemotherapy alone for treatment of HER2-positive advanced gastric or gastro-oesophageal junction cancer (ToGA): a phase 3, open-label, randomised controlled trial. Lancet 2010;376:687–97.

52. Available at: clinicaltrials.gov. Identifier NCT02120911. Accessed January 20, 2016.

53. Rice TW, Mason DP, Murthy SC, et al. T2N0M0 esophageal cancer. J Thorac Cardiovasc Surg 2007;133:317–24.

54. Kountourakis P, Correa AM, Hofstetter WL, et al. Combined modality therapy of cT2N0M0 esophageal

cancer: the University of Texas M. D. Anderson Cancer Center experience. Cancer 2011;117:925–30.

55. Crabtree TD, Kosinski AS, Puri V, et al. Evaluation of the reliability of clinical staging of T2 N0 esophageal cancer: a review of the Society of Thoracic Surgeons database. Ann Thorac Surg 2013;96:382–90.

56. Crabtree TD, Yacoub WN, Puri V, et al. Endoscopic ultrasound for early stage esophageal adenocarcinoma: implications for staging and survival. Ann Thorac Surg 2011;91:1509–15.

57. Stiles BM, Mirza F, Coppolino A, et al. Clinical T2-T3N0M0 esophageal cancer: the risk of node positive disease. Ann Thorac Surg 2011;92:491–6.

58. Zhang JQ, Hooker CM, Brock MV, et al. Neoadjuvant chemoradiation therapy is beneficial for clinical

stage T2 N0 esophageal cancer patients due to inaccurate preoperative staging. Ann Thorac Surg 2012;93:429–35.

59. Speicher PJ, Ganapathi AM, Englum BR, et al. Induction therapy does not improve survival for clinical stage T2N0 esophageal cancer. J Thorac Oncol 2014;9:1195.

60. Martin JT, Worni M, Zwischenberger JB, et al. The role of radiation therapy in resected T2 N0 esophageal cancer: a population-based analysis. Ann Thorac Surg 2013;95:453–8.

61. Smith GL, Smith BD, Buchholz TA, et al. Patterns of care and locoregional treatment outcomes in older esophageal cancer patients: The SEER-Medicare Cohort. Int J Radiat Oncol Biol Phys 2009;74:482–9.

The Evolution and Current Utility of Esophageal Stent Placement for the Treatment of Acute Esophageal Perforation

Argenis Herrera, MD[a], Richard K. Freeman, MD, MBA[b],*

KEYWORDS

- Esophageal perforation • Esophageal stent placement • Hybrid treatment strategy

KEY POINTS

- As part of a hybrid treatment strategy, including surgical drainage of infected spaces, enteral nutrition, and aggressive supportive care, esophageal stent placement has produced results that can exceed those of traditional surgical repair.

INTRODUCTION

The use of an esophageal stent for the treatment of an acute esophageal perforation was rarely reported or discussed before 2001. As discussed in this article, this is when advances in biomaterial allowed a new generation of stents to be manufactured that combined a nonpermeable covering, radial force sufficient to occlude a transmural esophageal injury, and improved removability. These developments set the stage for the use of an esophageal stent as part of an approach for the treatment of an acute esophageal perforation that eliminated the need for direct primary repair and its significant failure rate. Esophageal stent placement for the treatment of esophageal perforation or failed operative repair also had the potential to minimize the need for esophageal resection and diversion. This review summarizes the modern history of esophageal stent use in the treatment of esophageal perforation as well as the evidenced-based recommendations for the use of esophageal stent placement in the treatment of acute esophageal perforation.

HISTORY

The use of an endoluminal esophageal stent to treat esophageal stenosis, fistulae, and leaks is not a new concept for the thoracic surgeon. Esophageal intubation has been used since the nineteenth century when Symonds[1] in 1887 described the first successful experience with prostheses made of ivory and silver. In 1914, Guisez[2] was the first to place esophageal "tubes" to palliate esophageal obstructions under direct vision. Ten years later, Soutter[3] published his results using metallic tubes with a rubber funnel. Coyas[4] subsequently designed a plastic tube with metallic rings of equal diameter, which was better tolerated by patients with malignant dysphagia.

In more recent times, Mousseau and colleagues,[5] Atkinson and colleagues,[6] and Ferguson developed devices for esophageal intubation. Celestin,[7] modifying a French design by Mousseau and Barbin, developed a polythene stent for inoperable malignant strictures that was successful in maintaining oral intake. However, difficulty with

Disclosures: None.
[a] Department of Surgery, St Vincent Hospital, 8433 Harcourt Road, Indianapolis, IN 46260, USA; [b] Division of Thoracic and Cardiovascular Surgery, St Vincent Hospital, 8433 Harcourt Road, Indianapolis, IN 46260, USA
* Corresponding author.
E-mail address: Richard.Freeman@StVincent.org

Thorac Surg Clin 26 (2016) 305–314
http://dx.doi.org/10.1016/j.thorsurg.2016.04.012

insertion, migration, and extraction limited the use of these prostheses.

Taking advantage of the technology used to make endovascular stents, self-expanding metallic esophageal stents became available in the 1990s. These stents are woven, knitted, or laser-cut metallic mesh designed to exert self-expansive forces up to a fixed diameter. The metallic part is most often a steel alloy such as Elgiloy or nitinol. Elgiloy (cobalt, nickel, and chromium) is corrosion resistant and able to generate high radial pressures, whereas nitinol (nickel and titanium) allows more flexibility with less radial forces.[8,9]

Self-expanding metal stents offered the advantages of being inserted with flexible esophagoscopy, required significantly less esophageal dilatation, had a lower rate of migration, and provided improved palliation for malignant esophageal strictures and malignant tracheoesophageal fistulae.[10,11] However, there continued to be a reluctance to place these prostheses in the esophagus of a patient for conditions other than palliative therapy for a malignancy because of the potential esophageal damage associated with extraction, including reports of irreparable, sometimes life-threatening, fistulae.

In order to minimize tumor ingrowth and its complications, a second generation of metallic stent designs incorporated a covering of silicone, polyurethane, or other polymers.[12] This modification offered the advantage of diminishing the amount of tumor ingrowth and fixation of the stent to the esophageal wall theoretically at the cost of higher migration rates. In an attempt to minimize migration, metallic stents are also manufactured partially covered with a margin of 1.5 cm on the proximal and distal ends to optimize purchase of the esophageal wall.[13,14]

The next step in the evolution of esophageal stent biomaterials was the ability to produce an occlusive plastic prosthesis coated with silicone. This design has resulted in an esophageal stent with ease of insertion, a minimal requirement for esophageal dilation, and the ability to form an occlusive seal within the lumen of the esophagus.[15] A distinct advantage of these nonmetallic endoprostheses is also their ability to be removed or replaced even after long periods of time without damaging the esophagus. However, these stents are associated with a higher incidence of migration.[16]

The ability to easily place and remove a covered, occlusive stent in the esophagus led some investigators to implant these stents in select patients as a temporary measure to treat intrathoracic anastomotic leaks following esophagogastrostomy and acute perforations. Segalin and colleagues[16] and Roy-Choudhury and colleagues[17] were among the first to report the successful treatment of an esophageal perforation or an anastomotic leak using a self-expanding metal stent, respectively.

EARLY IMPLEMENTATION

Several other investigators reported their initial experiences treating acute perforations or anastomotic leaks between 2000 and 2005. Success rates in these series varied significantly as do the frequencies of stent migration, mortality, and healing. The variability in results is not unexpected given the lack of treatment protocols among investigators, the evolutionary nature of the technique during this period, and the diversity of stents used. Pleural drainage and enteral nutrition are noticeably absent as a consistent part of the treatment protocol.

Between 2005 and 2011, several series were reported containing at least 10 acute perforation patients treated with esophageal stent placement. Johnsson and colleagues[18] in 2005 and Fischer and colleagues[19] in 2006 reported 20 and 15 esophageal perforation patients, respectively, treated with self-expanding metal stents. Johnsson reported a 95% sealing rate for the perforation but only a 77% rate of healing. Fisher and colleagues realized a 100% rate of sealing the perforation and ultimate healing. Seven patients in this series developed an empyema requiring further intervention.

The evolution of esophageal stent use in the authors' practice began in patients who either were exceedingly high risk for the transthoracic repair of an esophageal leak or had undergone a previous operative repair that failed. The authors found this technique to be beneficial in these complex patients and reported their initial experience in 2007.[20] In this series, 21 patients who had undergone at least one failed operative repair of a chronic esophageal leak had a silicone-coated plastic stent placed in an attempt to seal the fistula without further surgery, resulting in 95% of these leaks being sealed without further surgery.

The encouraging results of this initial investigation led the authors to consider whether endoluminal esophageal stenting would be superior to primary operative repair in acute esophageal perforations. Recognizing the traditional goals of operative therapy for an esophageal perforation, they designed a hybrid treatment protocol that included operative or percutaneous drainage of infected spaces, the establishment of enteral nutrition, along with esophageal stet placement. They also thought it was important for the thoracic surgeon to be involved in these patients' care even when no surgery was required.

The authors next report of 17 patients with an acute iatrogenic esophageal perforation treated using this hybrid strategy, also in 2007, found that the perforation was sealed in 16 (94%) patients, with 82% resuming oral intake within 72 hours.[21] Stent migration occurred in 3 patients (18%). Mean hospital length of stay was 8 days (median 5 days), and there were no mortalities.

The authors then assessed the viability of using an esophageal stent in the treatment of a more difficult population of patients: those suffering a spontaneous esophageal perforation or Boerhaave syndrome. Reported in 2009, this series of 19 patients found that 17 patients (89%) sealed their perforation following stent placement.[22] Fifteen patients (79%) resumed oral intake within 72 hours of stent placement. Four patients (21%) had at least one episode of stent migration requiring repositioning or replacement. Again, no mortalities resulted in this patient series.

During this time period, other centers were gaining experience treating esophageal perforation with stenting as well. In 2009, Leers and colleagues[23] reported a series of 15 patients treated with self-expanding metal stents, achieving a success rate of 87% without further intervention. van Heel and colleagues[24] also reported a series of 33 patients with an esophageal perforation treated with a variety of stent types in 2010. Despite the stent sealing the perforation in 32 (97%) patients, 4 (12%) patients eventually required esophagectomy because of a recurrent leak or complications of removing the stent. In 2011, D'Cunha and colleagues[25] reported the University of Minnesota's experience with 37 patients, 15 of whom were treated for perforation. This study showed the value of a learning curve in the treatment of these patients and confirmed the hybrid approach of endoluminal stent placement with aggressive surgical drainage of infected spaces to be safe and effective in the treatment of acute esophageal perforation.

Over the last 5 years, the technique of esophageal stent placement for acute esophageal perforation has become more commonly used. As with any technique, the dissemination of this treatment strategy has allowed for continued innovation as well as some undesirable modifications. Ignoring the traditional goals of treatment of an esophageal perforation, some have chosen to use an esophageal stent as monotherapy for an esophageal perforation. Reports exist of multiple covered and uncovered stents being placed in patients with an esophageal perforation with continued mediastinal soilage without ever sealing the leak or draining infected spaces.[26,27] Such endeavors have predictably failed. Some investigators have also reported life-threatening vascular fistulas following lengthy stent dwell times.

The authors sought to address each of these reported concerns in 2 investigations. The first was an analysis of stent failures. Reviewing 187 patients who underwent stent placement, 4 factors were associated with an increase rate of failure: an injury greater than 6 cm in length, and injury that traversed the gastroesophageal junction or proximal cervical esophagus or was associated with a leak in the gastric conduit in esophagectomy patients.[28] Also emphasized was the need to recognize stent treatment failure early and move to a traditional operative repair to avoid the complications of mediastinitis and need for esophagectomy or esophageal diversion.

The authors' esophageal stenting experience was also reviewed in an attempt to determine the optimal time for esophageal stent removal.[29] Increased rates of complications were realized in patients whose stent was left in place for more than 4 weeks when treating an acute perforation or longer than 2 weeks when treating an anastomotic leak. Leaks that persisted beyond these time intervals were evaluated for surgical repair or a modification of stent therapy.

As mentioned, additional beneficial uses for the new generation of esophageal stenting have been recognized as familiarity with the current generation of esophageal stents has increased. Intrathoracic anastomotic leak following esophagogastrostomy remains a morbid complication of esophagectomy. However, several groups have shown that esophageal stent placement for such leaks are safe and effective treatment while avoiding reoperation or diversion in the vast majority of cases. The authors' group reported a series of 17 patients, most of whom were treated with preoperative chemotherapy and radiation therapy, in which all of the anastomotic leaks were sealed with esophageal stent placement.[30] Stent migration occurred in only 3 patients and was treated exclusively with endoscopic removal and replacement (18%).

Keeling and colleagues,[31] when reporting their results in primary surgical repair of esophageal perforation patients, discussed their successful novel use of an esophageal stent in 2 patients whose leak persisted. The authors subsequently reviewed their experience in patients treated with surgical repair who continued to experience a significant leak.[32] In a series of 32 such patients, esophageal stent placement was able to "rescue" the initial repair and allowed healing in 29 (93%) patients without further operative intervention.

CURRENT STATE

It is the authors' current practice to consider esophageal stent placement for any esophageal perforation, fistula, or anastomotic leak (**Fig. 1**). This current practice is regardless of the duration of the perforation or fistula before treatment or whether a previous operative repair has been performed. Included are patients who have a relatively large esophageal diameter and patients with systemic manifestations of infection related to their esophageal injury.

The authors have also successfully treated acute perforations and fistulae of the esophagus in the setting of an esophageal malignancy. Although generally considered an indication for esophagectomy rather than operative repair, esophageal injury or fistula in the setting of malignancy will often seal with endoluminal stent placement. Systemic chemotherapy and/or radiation therapy is discontinued for a 2-week period but can then be restarted.

Exclusion Criteria

As with any technique, there are some relative contraindications to this form of treatment. Long segment perforations of the esophagus (>6 cm) and esophageal injuries recognized during another operative procedure or in a patient that will require an immediate thoracotomy for an associated injury are generally treated with a traditional operative repair. Acute injuries of the cervical esophagus are also generally treated with operative repair because the operative approach is better tolerated, the rate of success is higher than intrathoracic repair, and it is recognized that most patients cannot tolerate a stent that lies proximal to the cricopharyngeus muscle. However, the authors have had success treating chronic fistulae of the cervical esophagus using an esophageal stent in select patients.

In the case of an intrathoracic anastomotic leak following esophagectomy, a near complete dehiscence of the anastomosis or focal or generalized conduit necrosis is not treated by esophageal stent placement for obvious reasons. Similarly, esophagectomy patients whose foregut continuity was reestablished with a conduit other than the stomach who experience an anastomotic leak have not undergone esophageal stent placement in the authors' practice. The endoluminal stent size required to seal the larger-caliber esophageal side of an anastomotic leak can result in necrosis of a jejunal conduit, whereas the potential for significant complications related to stent migration is increased if the colon was used for reconstruction.

Stent Placement Technique

The presence of an esophageal perforation, fistula, or anastomotic leak is documented and localized by a Gastrografin and/or barium esophagram before entering the operating room (**Fig. 2**). To be considered a significant leak eligible for treatment other than observation, contrast should be seen leaving the lumen of the esophagus into the mediastinum, pleural, or peritoneal space. In addition, all patients being considered for stent placement undergo computer-aided tomographic imaging of the neck, chest, and abdomen to identify areas of secondary infection requiring intervention (**Fig. 3**).

All esophageal stents are placed in the operating room using general anesthesia and fluoroscopy by a thoracic surgeon following flexible esophagoscopy. The purposes of esophagoscopy are to localize the esophageal leak and decide which size stent should be used (**Fig. 4**). The authors' approach has been to oversize the stent both in length and in diameter. This oversizing has had a beneficial effect on stent migration and the ability to seal a leak relatively quickly. The authors generally use a 21- to 25-mm-diameter stent in the longest length possible without crossing the gastroesophageal junction or the Arytenoid fold of the posterior oropharynx. They have not found it beneficial to routinely place more than one stent in the esophagus in an attempt to seal a perforation, fistula, or anastomotic leak.

They also place a percutaneous endoscopic gastrostomy just before esophageal stent placement if the patient does not have another form of enteral access and has not undergone esophagectomy. This percutaneous endoscopic gastrostomy can be placed to gravity drainage for the first 24 hours, eliminating the need for a nasogastric tube with feedings initiated thereafter. If a percutaneous gastrostomy cannot be placed, a laparoscopic tube jejunostomy is performed.

The esophageal stent is then placed by marking the proximal and distal landmarks pertinent to deploying the stent viewed endoscopically using fluoroscopy (**Fig. 5**). Specifically, the proximal and distal extent of the esophageal leak and the gastroesophageal junction are marked with a radiopaque object. A guidewire specific to the stent chosen for use is then placed through the endoscope into the stomach. The stent is then moved into position using fluoroscopy and deployed. Flexible esophagoscopy is then used to confirm that the stent has properly deployed.

The stent can be easily moved to a more proximal position using an endoscopic grasper, endoscopy, and fluoroscopy, if required. However, if the

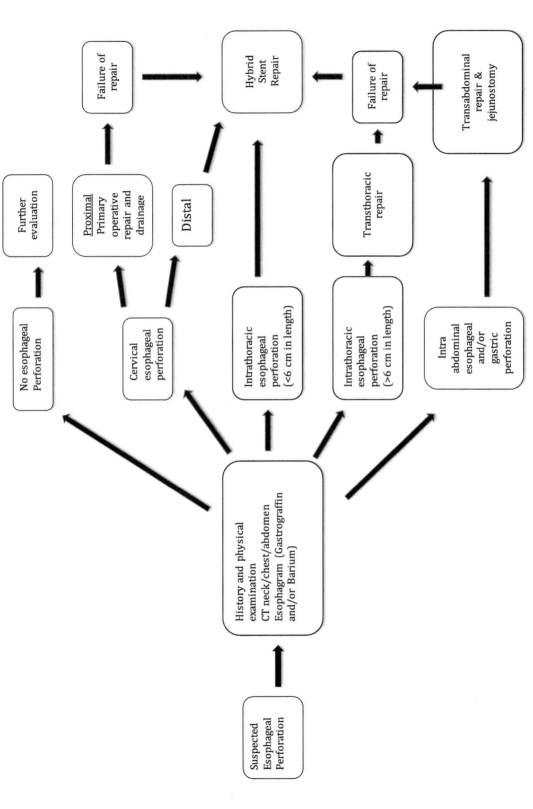

Fig. 1. Current algorithm for esophageal stent use.

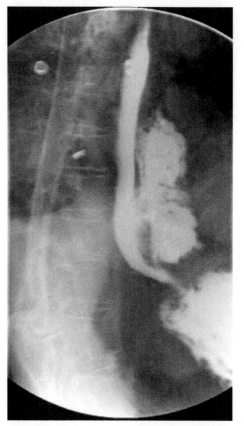

Fig. 2. Contrast esophagram displaying a midthoracic esophageal perforation.

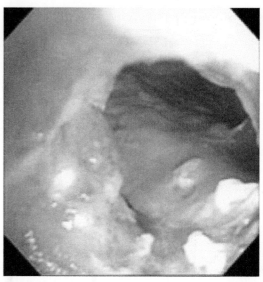

Fig. 4. Endoscopic view of an acute esophageal perforation.

stent is too proximal after deployment, it will likely need to be removed and replaced to prevent further injury to the esophagus. If the stent does not open completely after its deployment, a pneumatic esophageal dilatation balloon can be used to expand it. However, after 12 to 24 hours, almost all such wrinkles will completely expand without further intervention.

The authors have not found it beneficial to perform a contrast study at the time of stent placement. Endoscopy following stent placement yields a better assessment of stent position and deployment in relation to the esophageal leak (Fig. 6). The stent also requires some time to equilibrate to body temperature, maximally expand, and seal the perforation. The authors prefer to perform a contrast esophagram 48 to 72 hours following stent placement, as described later.

Adequate drainage of infected areas is achieved during the same anesthesia by either video-assisted thoracoscopy, laparoscopy, or image-guided percutaneous drainage. Such procedures are planned based on the preoperative imaging studies and findings at the time of endoscopy. The authors do not routinely perform a tracheostomy in these patients unless they have already required prolonged mechanical ventilation to reduce the possibility of tracheoesophageal fistula formation with prostheses in both the esophagus and the trachea.

As with many surgical procedures, the care of the patient following esophageal stent placement is just as important as the performance of the procedure itself. The authors think it is important that

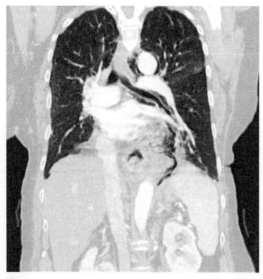

Fig. 3. Computer-aided tomographic imaging of the chest following an esophageal perforation.

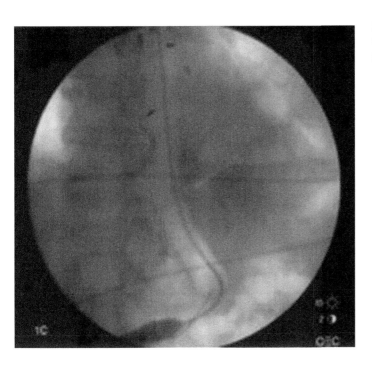

Fig. 5. Fluoroscopic image of an esophageal stent placement for acute perforation.

the thoracic surgeon direct the care of these patients just as if they had undergone an operative repair. This treatment is not only important in making sure patients who fail stent therapy receive timely operative intervention but also essential in determining that all associated areas of intrathoracic or intra-abdominal infection are adequately treated.

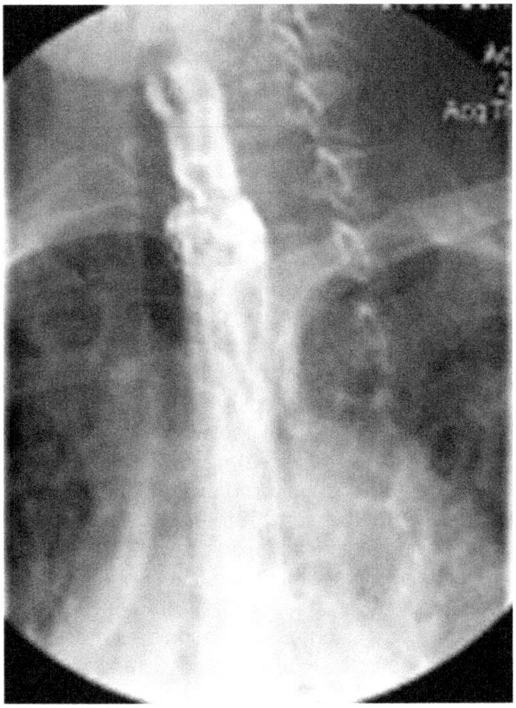

Similarly, the systemic inflammatory response and/or sepsis experienced by some of these patients require that they be cared for with the same vigilance as if they had undergone an operative repair, including appropriate fluid resuscitation, prophylactic antimicrobial therapy adjusted by culture data, and cardiopulmonary support administered in a critical care environment. Especially important is the immediate initiation of nutrition, preferably via an enteral route.

Patients with persistent or recurrent fevers, organ failure, or leukocytosis undergo computer-aided tomographic imaging of the neck, chest, and abdomen every 48 to 72 hours to look for evidence of surgically treatable infection.[6] If identified, such infection must be aggressively treated. It is the authors' preference to perform such procedures in a minimally invasive fashion, when possible.

Leak occlusion is confirmed by a contrast esophagram a minimum of 24 hours after stent placement or when the patient is able to participate in the examination (see Fig. 5). In the absence of a continued leak, an oral diet specific to the esophageal stent is initiated. This diet is essentially a "mechanical soft" diet that excludes bread and meat in an attempt to minimize stent migration. Enteral feeding is continued until the patient can

Fig. 6. Esophagram 48 hours after esophageal stent placement for acute perforation.

consume sufficient calories to maintain their nutritional parameters.

Patients who begin an oral diet continue to be treated with a daily proton pump inhibitor and multivitamin to maximize the potential for healing of the esophageal injury. Aspiration precautions are observed with each patient being evaluated for the ability to swallow at the bedside. Most patients after the procedure pain can be managed initially with patient-controlled analgesia using a short-acting opioid. Patients are usually discharged with an oral narcotic elixir, if required. In contrast to the rare patient with benign disease who experiences pain severe enough to require stent removal, the authors have not removed stents placed for perforation, fistula, or anastomotic leak because of intractable pain.

Stent migration does occur when esophageal stent placement is used to treat patients with an esophageal perforation, fistula, or anastomotic leak. Techniques previously described can minimize the frequency of its occurrence. However, the thoracic surgeon should be vigilant of its possibility. Most patients can be assessed for stent migration using a chest roentgenogram. If migration is suspected, endoscopy in the operating room with everything required to reposition or replace the stent should occur as soon as possible. During endoscopy, the site of the esophageal leak or injury should be carefully inspected because migration can be a sign that the leak has been sealed. The authors do not exchange an esophageal stent unless migration not amenable to repositioning has occurred or if the integrity of the stent is compromised.

It is the intention to remove all patients' esophageal stents following a sufficient amount of time to allow the leak to seal. This removal is individualized for each patient, taking into consideration the resolution of any indications of systemic infection. Stent removal is also carried out in the operating room under general anesthesia. Flexible esophagoscopy is performed before and after stent removal, and an esophagram is performed before oral intake is resumed.

The authors' experience has led them to remove stents much earlier than they did in their initial series due to a better understanding of how these leaks seal and then heal, with adherence to adjacent structures creating a watertight seal followed by eventual tissue in-growth and repair. Several reports of significant complications related to indwelling esophageal stents including tracheoesophageal fistulae, aortoesophageal fistulae, and bowel obstruction resulting from stent migration have also prompted them to routinely consider stent removal after 10 to 14 days.

Any measure of success in treating patients with an esophageal injury that they have obtained stems from the authors' adherence to several basic principles: management directed by a thoracic surgeon, early diagnosis, confirmation of sealing of the esophageal discontinuity after stent placement, and drainage of pleura cavity with simultaneous percutaneous endoscopic gastrostomy tube for early enteral nutrition, while the patient is managed in the intensive care unit. Intravenous antibiotic coverage is started early.

The thoracic surgeon must be involved in the care decisions for patients with esophageal perforation. This involved is important both to identify contraindications for stent placement, in which immediate operative repair is undertaken, and to rapidly identify and treat stent failures. It is also important to ensure that these patients receive the level of care their condition requires, including aggressive antimicrobial and nutritional therapy, surveillance for continued areas of infection, and critical care support.

Outcomes

Any analysis of the effectiveness of esophageal stent placement must be made in the context of the application of the technique and in comparison to the available treatment alternatives. The authors feel strongly that esophageal stent placement as monotherapy for esophageal perforation is inadequate and does not recognize the traditional goals of therapy for a patient with an esophageal perforation; a principle confirmed by a recent literature review by Dasari and colleagues.[31] Therefore, it is not surprising to see results in some series or isolated case reports that are not comparable to a hybrid treatment protocol that emphasizes drainage of infected spaces, enteral nutrition, and early recognition of persistent leak with stent revision or operative repair.

Despite advances in surgical technique, critical care, and antimicrobial therapy, surgical repair continues to be associated with a postoperative leak rate reported between 30% and 40% at experienced centers.[32,33] The reported rate of successful stent use in esophageal perforation is at least comparable if not superior to these results without the need for thoracotomy. Stent use also provides a rescue mechanism for failed operative repair and has nearly eliminated the need for esophagectomy or esophageal diversion in the authors' practice. Stent use may also reduce the incidence of long-term esophageal stricture when compared with operative repair.

Like any technique, esophageal stent use for acute perforation does have its associated morbidities. The principal complication associated with stent use remains stent migration. The use of an esophageal stent also commits the patient to a return to surgery for stent removal and/or revision if migration does occur. Last, rarely reported fatal complications have been reported from vascular fistulae with what are now considered excessive stent dwell times.

It is doubtful for several reasons that a randomized trial between stent placement and operative repair for acute esophageal perforation will occur in the near future, not the least of which is the possible lack or equipoise between the 2 patient cohorts based on recent literature. However, comparisons can be made between the 2 treatment groups. In 2014, the authors reported a propensity matched comparison of patients treated at multiple institutions with either an esophageal stent or an operative repair following the recognition of an acute esophageal perforation.[34] In these well-matched groups, the esophageal stent cohort realized significant differences in morbidity (4% vs 43%; P = .02), mean length of stay (6 vs 11 days; P = .0007), time to oral intake (3 vs 8 days; P = .0004), and cost ($91,000 vs $142,000; P<.0001) were identified in the esophageal stent cohort when compared with patients receiving surgical repair. Ben-David and colleagues[35] reported similar findings in a recently published single-center experience.

Although the authors have been pleased with the results of endoluminal esophageal stent placement for the treatment of esophageal injuries, there are significant questions that remain to be answered. These queries include comparing different types of stents in a prospective fashion and assessing the results of this technique in multiple centers using a common treatment protocol. The authors continue to investigate the use of esophageal stents for esophageal perforation, fistula, or anastomotic leak as well as less common benign and malignant disorders of the esophagus. It is their belief that with continued investigation and refinement, esophageal stent placement will become a more integral part of the thoracic surgeon's armamentarium when caring for patients with acute and chronic diseases of the esophagus.

REFERENCES

1. Symonds CJ. The treatment of malignant stricture of the oesophagus by tubage or permanent catheterism. BMJ 1887;1:870–81.
2. Guisez J. De l'intubation caouchoutee oesophienne. Presse Med 1914;22:85.
3. Soutter HS. A method of intubating the esophagus for malignant stricture. BMJ 1924;1:782.
4. Coyas A. Palliative intubation in carcinoma of the oesophagus. Lancet 1955;2:647–9.
5. Mousseau M, Le Forestier J, Barbin J, et al. Place de 1'intubation a demeure dans le traitement palliative du cancer de 1'oesophage. Arch Mai Appar Digest 1956;45:208–16.
6. Atkinson M, Ferguson R, Ogilvie AL. Management of malignant dysphagia by intubation at endoscopy. JRSM 1979;72:894–7.
7. Celestin LR. Permanent intubation in inoperable cancer of the oesophagus and cardia: a new tube. Ann R Coll Surg Engl 1959;25:165–70.
8. Chan ACW, Shin FG, Lam YH, et al. A comparison study on physical properties of self-expandable esophageal metal stents. Gastrointest Endosc 1999;49:462–6.
9. Schmassmann A, Meyenberger C, Knuchel J, et al. Self-expanding metal stents in malignant esophageal obstruction: a comparison between two stent types. Am J Gastroenterol 1997;92:400–6.
10. Ell C, Hochberger J, May A, et al. Coated and uncoated self-expanding metal stents for malignant stenosis in the upper GI tract: preliminary clinical experiences with Wallstents. Am J Gastroenterol 1994; 1994(89):1496–500.
11. Nelson D, Silvis S, Ansel H. Management of a tracheoesophageal fistula with a silicone-covered self-expanding metal stent. Gastrointest Endosc 1994;40:497–9.
12. Ramirez F, Dennert B, Zierer S, et al. Esophageal self-expandable metallic stents–indications, practice, techniques, and complications: results of a national survey. Gastrointest Endosc 1997;45:360–4.
13. Saxon R, Morrison K, Lakin P, et al. Malignant esophageal obstruction and esophagorespiratory fistula: palliation with a polyethylene-covered Z-stent. Radiology 1997;202:349–54.
14. Decker P, Lippler J, Decker D, et al. Use of the Polyflex stent in the palliative therapy of esophageal carcinoma: results in 14 cases and review of the literature. Surg Endosc 2001;15(12):1444–7.
15. Gelbmann C, Ratiu N, Rath H, et al. Use of self-expandable plastic stents for the treatment of esophageal perforations and symptomatic anastomotic leaks. Endoscopy 2004;36:695–9.
16. Segalin A, Bonavina L, Lazzerini M, et al. Endoscopic management of inveterate esophageal perforations and leaks. Surg Endosc 1996;10:928–32.
17. Roy-Choudhury SH, Nicholson AA, Wedgwood KR, et al. Symptomatic malignant gastroesophageal anastomotic leak: management with covered metallic esophageal stents. AJR Am J Roentgenol 2001;176:161–5.
18. Johnsson E, Lundell L, Liedman B. Sealing of esophageal perforation or ruptures with expandable

metallic stents: a prospective controlled study on treatment efficacy and limitations. Dis Esophagus 2005;18:262–6.

19. Fischer A, Thomusch O, Benz S, et al. Nonoperative treatment of 15 benign esophageal perforations with self-expandable covered metal stents. Ann Thorac Surg 2006;81:467–72.

20. Freeman RK, Ascioti AJ, Wozniak TC. Postoperative esophageal leak management with the Polyflex esophageal stent. J Thorac Cardiovasc Surg 2007;133:333–8.

21. Freeman RK, Van Woerkom JM, Ascioti AJ. Esophageal stent placement for the treatment of iatrogenic intrathoracic esophageal perforation. Ann Thorac Surg 2007;83:2003–7.

22. Freeman RK, Van Woerkom JM, Vyverberg A, et al. Esophageal stent placement for the treatment of spontaneous esophageal perforations. Ann Thorac Surg 2009;88:194–8.

23. Leers JM, Vivaldi C, Schafer H, et al. Endoscopic therapy for esophageal perforation or anastomotic leak with a self-expandable metallic stent. Surg Endosc 2009;23:2258–62.

24. van Heel NC, Haringsma J, Spaander MC, et al. Short-term esophageal stenting in the management of benign perforations. Am J Gastroenterol 2010;105:1515–20.

25. D'Cunha J, Rueth NM, Groth SS, et al. Esophageal stents for anastomotic leaks and perforations. J Thorac Cardiovasc Surg 2011;142:39–46.

26. Odell JA, DeVault KR. Extended stent usage for persistent esophageal leak: should there be limits? Ann Thorac Surg 2010;90:1707–8.

27. Whitelock D, Maddaus M, Andrade R, et al. Gastroaortic fistula: a rare and lethal complication of esophageal stenting after esophagectomy. J Thorac Cardiovasc Surg 2010;140:e49–50.

28. Freeman RK, Ascioti AJ, Giannini T, et al. An analysis of unsuccessful esophageal stent placements for esophageal perforation, fistula or anastomotic leak. Ann Thorac Surg 2012;94:959–65.

29. Freeman RK, Ascioti AJ, Dake M, et al. An assessment of the optimal time for removal of esophageal stents used in the treatment of an esophageal anastomotic leak or perforation. Ann Thorac Surg 2015;100(2):422–8.

30. Freeman RK, Ascioti AJ, Dake M, et al. An analysis of esophageal stent placement for persistent leak after the operative repair of intrathoracic esophageal perforation. Ann Thorac Surg 2014;97:1715–20.

31. Dasari BV, Neely D, Kennedy A, et al. The role of esophageal stents in the management of esophageal anastomotic leaks and benign esophageal perforations. Ann Surg 2014;259:852–60.

32. Keeling WB, Miller DL, Lam GT, et al. Low mortality after treatment for esophageal perforation: a single-center experience. Ann Thorac Surg 2010;90:1669–73.

33. Wright CD, Mathisen DJ, Wain JC, et al. Reinforced primary repair of thoracic esophageal perforation. Ann Thorac Surg 1995;60:245–8.

34. Freeman RK, Herrera A, Ascioti AJ, et al. A propensity-matched comparison of cost and outcomes following esophageal stent placement or primary surgical repair for esophageal perforation. J Thorac Cardiovasc Surg 2015;149:1550–5.

35. Ben-David K, Behrns K, Hochwald S, et al. Esophageal perforation management using a multidisciplinary minimally invasive treatment algorithm. J Am Coll Surg 2014;218:768–74.

Lymph Node Dissection and Pulmonary Metastasectomy

Smita Sihag, MD, Ashok Muniappan, MD*

KEYWORDS

- Lymph node • Lung • Metastasectomy

KEY POINTS

- Intrathoracic lymph node involvement is associated with decreased survival after pulmonary metastasectomy. The data are most convincing for colorectal and renal cell cancers.
- The number of lymph nodes involved may have greater prognostic value than lymph node station involved. There is no clear survival difference between patients with N1 versus N2 nodal disease.
- Risk factors for intrathoracic lymph node metastases include enlarged or hypermetabolic nodes, large solitary metastases requiring anatomic resection, and multiple metastatic lesions. Mediastinal lymph node assessment should be considered in these patients, especially if findings may lead to further adjuvant therapy.
- There is limited evidence as to whether mediastinal lymphadenectomy leads to improved survival in patients undergoing pulmonary metastasectomy.
- The level of evidence to support any recommendations is low because the literature available for review is exclusively retrospective.

INTRODUCTION

According to the landmark report of the International Registry of Lung Metastases (IRLM), which included 5206 patients, the overall survival after pulmonary metastasectomy is 36% at 5 years, 26% at 10 years, and 22% at 15 years.[1] Given these encouraging findings and generally limited potential for long-term survival with standard systemic therapy for isolated pulmonary metastases, metastasectomy is considered whenever possible. The primary variables affecting survival after metastasectomy are derived from the IRLM and other single-center retrospective studies, and to date, there have been no randomized trials evaluating the effect of pulmonary metastasectomy on survival. The registry revealed that patients with germ cell tumors have the

highest 5-year survival rate at 68%, whereas those with melanoma have the lowest at 21%. Fewer metastases, complete resection, and longer disease-free interval before pulmonary metastasis are all associated with improved survival in patients undergoing metastasectomy. The registry, however, does not offer insight on the impact and relevance of mediastinal or hilar lymph node involvement. Metastasis to mediastinal or hilar lymph nodes was identified in 5% of patients (11% of germ cell tumors, 8% of melanomas, 6% of epithelial tumors, and 2% of sarcomas). Mediastinal lymph node sampling was performed at the discretion of the surgeon and was not routine. Although no survival difference was found with respect to presence or absence of nodal disease in the registry, incomplete resection was

Disclosures: The authors have no financial disclosures.
Department of Thoracic Surgery, Massachusetts General Hospital, Harvard Medical School, 55 Fruit Street, Blake 1570, Boston, MA 02114, USA
* Corresponding author.
E-mail address: amuniappan@partners.org

Thorac Surg Clin 26 (2016) 315–323
http://dx.doi.org/10.1016/j.thorsurg.2016.04.004

more likely in patients with positive nodes (27% vs 11%). The prognostic relevance of N1 and N2 nodal disease in the setting of pulmonary metastases has remained a topic of investigation in several subsequent studies.

Systematic mediastinal lymphadenectomy or sampling is routinely performed in the setting of primary neoplasms of the lung, including adenocarcinoma, squamous cell carcinoma (SCC), and neuroendocrine tumors. Controversy exists, however, surrounding the need for mediastinal lymph node assessment at pulmonary metastasectomy. Based on a survey of 146 surgeons from the European Society of Thoracic Surgeons, 55% indicated that they regularly sample mediastinal lymph nodes at the time of metastasectomy, whereas 33% avoided nodal dissection.[2] Although approximately 65% of surgeons considered mediastinal nodal metastasis to be an absolute contraindication, only 4% of surgeons regularly performed mediastinoscopy prior to metastasectomy. This article reviews the evidence for prognostic significance of intrathoracic lymph node status by origin of primary tumor. The identification of positive mediastinal lymph nodes may guide further management of metastatic disease to the lung in terms of adjuvant systemic therapy, timing of administration, and extent of pulmonary resection.

INTRATHORACIC LYMPH NODE INVOLVEMENT AND ISOLATED PULMONARY METASTASIS BY PRIMARY TUMOR HISTOLOGY
Colorectal Carcinoma

Approximately half of all patients with colorectal cancer develop metastatic disease at some point in the course of their disease. Increasingly, patients undergo pulmonary and hepatic metastasectomy, the primary sites of metastasis.[3] Patients with untreated stage IV disease have a median survival of only 8 months, whereas treatment with 5-fluorouracil–based chemotherapy prolongs median survival to 24 to 28 months.[4] In contrast, patients who undergo complete resection of pulmonary metastases of colorectal cancer have a 5-year survival of up to 60%.[5] Prognostic factors that have been found to affect survival include carcinoembryonic antigen level, disease-free interval before development of metastases, number of metastases, and the completeness of resection of all metastatic disease.

The incidence of intrathoracic lymph node metastases at the time of pulmonary metastasectomy for colorectal cancer is reported to be in the range of 12% to 44%.[3,6] The variability in the reported incidence of nodal involvement is related to heterogeneity in the burden of metastatic disease as well as inconsistent sampling or dissection of intrathoracic nodes. Intrathoracic lymph node metastasis in colorectal cancer is associated with decreased survival in numerous reports. In a retrospective study from the Mayo Clinic of 518 patients, of whom 319 underwent lymph node assessment, mediastinal lymph node involvement was identified in 40 patients (13%).[6] Of these 40 patients, 9 (23%) had N1 disease, and 31 (77%) had N2 disease. In this study, only lymph node size greater than 1 cm and fludeoxyglucose F 18 (FDG) avidity predicted the presence of lymph node metastases, whereas size, number, and location of pulmonary metastases did not. Furthermore, there was no correlation between location of the metastatic lesion and the lymph node station involved. Five-year survival was 48% in the negative lymph node group and 21% in the positive lymph node group. Although mediastinal lymph node involvement was a significant predictor of inferior survival in this study, long-term survival was possible in a few patients with N2-positive nodes.

Several studies suggest that the 5-year survival rate is approximately halved if intrathoracic lymph node involvement is identified in colorectal metastasis. In a retrospective analysis of 169 patients from Germany who underwent colorectal metastasectomy, 17% were found to have metastases to intrathoracic lymph nodes.[5] Lymph node sampling or regional lymphadenectomy were only performed, however, if lymph nodes appeared abnormal at intraoperative assessment. Five-year survival with positive lymph nodes was 19% as opposed to 42% in patients without nodal metastasis. There were no patients who survived 5 years in the presence of N2 or mediastinal metastasis. Another single-center retrospective report from France similarly observed diminished long-term survival in the setting of positive mediastinal lymph nodes, although they reported that 39% of patients with N1 or N2 metastases survived 5 years.[7] In a larger retrospective study of 320 patients at another French center, where routine lymphadenectomy was performed at the time of metastasectomy, 44% had positive intrathoracic lymph nodes.[3] Of these 140 patients, 91 (65%) had N1 disease, and 49 (35%) had N2 disease. Lymph node involvement was more likely in patients with multiple pulmonary metastases. Median length of survival in patients with positive lymph nodes was half that of patients without nodal metastases (42 months vs 94 months) but was still longer than expected for patients receiving systemic therapy alone for metastatic colorectal cancer. There was no significant difference in survival between those with N1 or N2 nodal involvement. In this study, a quarter of all patients with positive N2 nodal disease were found to have skip metastases, without evidence of N1 nodal involvement.

Although the distinction between N1 or N2 nodal involvement does not seem to be a meaningful predictor of survival, the lymph node ratio (number of lymph nodes involved divided by number of lymph nodes examined) may have prognostic value. In a follow-up study by Renaud and colleagues,[8] the average number of lymph nodes retrieved during systematic mediastinal lymph node dissection was 21 in 106 patients with nodal involvement; 66 patients had N1 disease and 40 patients had N2 disease. Regardless of lymph node station, lymph node ratio greater than 50% was associated with a significantly lower median survival (17 vs 30 months) as well as a higher risk of locoregional recurrence with an odds ratio of 2.75 ($P = .02$).

In addition to the number of lymph nodes involved, it seems that the location of the colorectal primary also affects the risk of metastasis and long-term survival. Lower and middle rectal cancers were associated with higher rates of intrathoracic nodal metastases compared with upper rectal and colon cancers (29% vs 16%).[4] Anatomic differences in lymphatic and venous drainage of middle and lower rectal cancers likely explain a greater propensity for intrathoracic nodal metastasis, which is associated with inferior survival. Greater attention to intrathoracic nodal assessment is probably warranted in middle and lower rectal tumors, because positive findings likely have an impact on prognostication and decision making regarding adjuvant therapies and extent of resection. Colon and upper third rectal tumors, on the other hand, are less likely to metastasize to intrathoracic nodes. In one study, all patients with fewer than 4 pulmonary metastases amenable to wedge resection and a colonic primary and who underwent routine lymph node dissection, no nodal disease was identified.[9] The investigators speculated that minimally invasive resections without aggressive nodal assessment may be adequate for these patients. Risk factors for intrathoracic lymph node metastases included rectal site of origin, multiple metastases to the lung, and the need for anatomic lung resection to achieve a negative margin.

Renal Cell Carcinoma

Renal cell carcinoma (RCC) metastases are poorly responsive to chemotherapy and radiotherapy, and currently no clinically proved adjuvant therapy is available after pulmonary metastasectomy. Whenever feasible, definitive surgical resection is the treatment of choice for isolated pulmonary metastases. Approximately 30% of patients with metastatic RCC to the lung have positive intrathoracic lymph nodes, with mediastinal involvement in half.[10] As in the case of colorectal cancer, multiple retrospective studies suggest that mediastinal and hilar lymph node metastasis discovered at pulmonary metastasectomy is a negative prognostic factor for survival.

In a large single-center study from Germany, of 110 patients who underwent pulmonary metastasectomy and routine intrathoracic lymph node dissection for RCC, 35% had histologically proved lymph node metastases.[11] The distribution of nodal stations involved were isolated N1 disease in 7%, isolated N2 disease in 16%, and combined N1 and N2 disease in 12% of patients. The incidence of lymph node metastasis was not affected by the number, size, or recurrence of pulmonary metastases nor did it correlate with lymph node status of the primary tumor. Patients without intrathoracic lymph node metastasis had considerably longer median survival (102.2 months vs 19.1 months). Patients with N2 nodal disease had slightly decreased median survival of 13.8 months compared with 19.1 months for patients with N1 nodal disease.

In a follow-up study, Meimarakis and colleagues[12] proposed a prognostic scoring system, the Munich score, to predict long-term survival after resection pulmonary RCC metastases. They enrolled 200 consecutive patients, 87% of whom underwent curative R0 pulmonary metastasectomy, and observed a median survival of 43 months. Complete hilar and mediastinal intrathoracic lymph node dissection was performed in 91 patients. Hilar or mediastinal nodal metastases were identified in 27 patients (30%). Multivariate analysis revealed that complete resection, size greater than 3 cm, positive nodal status of primary tumor, synchronous metastasis, pleural disease, and tumor infiltration of hilar or mediastinal lymph nodes as independent prognostic factors for survival. Median survival was reduced with intrathoracic nodal involvement (19 months vs 32 months).

The scoring system allowed them to stratify patients into 3 groups: low risk (1 risk factor, median survival 43 months), intermediate risk (2 risk factors, median survival 16 months), and high risk (3 risk factors, median survival 8 months) for poor survival. It is uncertain whether high-risk patients derived any benefit from pulmonary metastasectomy. The investigators speculated that high-risk patients may represent a select subgroup of patients with metastatic RCC that may benefit from systemic adjuvant therapy. Because intrathoracic nodal metastasis is one of the pillars of this scoring system and an important prognostic variable, routine mediastinal lymph node assessment seems advisable in patients undergoing pulmonary metastasectomy for metastatic RCC.

Exclusion of patients with RCC and intrathoracic nodal metastases from surgical resection of pulmonary metastases, however, is not supported in a review of 122 patients from 2 centers in France that specifically investigated this issue, particularly in the setting of N2 disease.[13] Although mediastinal and hilar lymph node involvement was identified as a significant prognostic factor, with median survival of 37 months as opposed to 107 months in patients without nodal disease, hilar or mediastinal location had no significant effect on survival, and N1 and N2 disease were prognostically equivalent. Although the number of node-positive patients was relatively small, this study demonstrated that long-term survival can be achieved in some patients despite intrathoracic nodal metastasis.

Sarcoma

The incidence of pulmonary metastasis is as high as 20% for osteogenic sarcoma and 40% for soft tissue sarcoma, and the lung is frequently the only site of distant metastasis. Even after aggressive surgical resection of pulmonary metastases, recurrence rates are as high as 50%.[14] Although systemic chemotherapy is of limited proven benefit in the treatment of metastatic sarcoma, retrospective studies have demonstrated a 5-year survival rate of close to 40% with pulmonary metastasectomy.[15]

The incidence of lymphatic metastases in the setting of sarcomatous pulmonary metastasis has not been precisely reported. Moreover, the role of thoracic lymph node dissection in metastatic sarcoma has not been studied separately, and available data are from studies that have combined patients with diverse primary tumor origins. Pfannschmidt and colleagues[16] reported their experience with 245 patients who underwent pulmonary metastasectomy with systematic and routine hilar and mediastinal lymph node dissection. In this series, 69 patients had pulmonary metastases secondary to osteogenic or soft-tissue sarcoma. The prevalence of lymph node involvement for patients with sarcoma was 20%, with N2 mediastinal involvement in 10%. No patients had both N1 and N2 disease in the sarcoma group, making the prevalence of noncontiguous nodal metastases highest in sarcoma, of all the tumor histologies examined. The median survival for metastasectomy for sarcoma was 47 months for node-negative patients, 18.3 months for patients with positive N1 nodes, and 22 months for patients with positive N2 nodes. Although there was a significant difference in survival between N0 and N+ patients ($P = .036$), survival was similar in patients with either N1 or N2 node involvement. Given the limited efficacy of systemic therapy for metastatic sarcoma, patients should not necessarily be excluded from metastasectomy solely for the reason of nodal involvement, because it seems some measure of disease control is achievable in well-selected patients.

Pfannschmidt and colleagues[17] also reported a separate subgroup analysis of 50 patients with pulmonary metastases from soft tissue sarcoma. They observed a 5-year survival rate of 53% with complete resection of metastatic disease. Neither disease-free interval, intrathoracic lymph node metastases, nor number of metastases, however, were found to be significant prognostic factors. Given the few reports concerning intrathoracic nodal metastasis in sarcoma, it is difficult to conclude whether or not mediastinal lymphadenectomy should be routinely performed in patients with sarcomatous pulmonary metastases for purposes of staging, prognostication, selection for alternative adjuvant therapies, or improving survival.

Germ Cell Tumors

For nonseminomatous germ cell tumors of testicular origin with normalization of tumor markers after induction cisplatin-based chemotherapy, resection of intrathoracic metastases with curative intent is standard treatment.[18] Long-term survival in this typically younger population is generally the best of all tumors that metastasize to the lung, even in the setting of mediastinal nodal disease. In a series of 52 patients who underwent pulmonary resection for intrathoracic metastases after cisplatin-based chemotherapy, overall 5-year survival was reported to be 76%.[19] Normalization of serum tumor markers prior to resection improved survival and may be related to completeness of resection, which is a significant prognostic factor for long-term survival. Systematic mediastinal and hilar lymph node dissection was performed in all but 4 patients, and nodal metastases were found in 33% of patients. Kesler and colleagues[20] found no difference in survival in patients undergoing resection of pulmonary or mediastinal metastases. They described their current surgical strategy for resecting pulmonary and mediastinal metastases; particularly important is the approach to the lower visceral mediastinal compartment, which is accessed typically at the time of the retroperitoneal lymph node dissection. Mediastinal lymph node metastases are resected completely with therapeutic intent, and there is no role for lymph node sampling.

Melanoma

Pulmonary metastasectomy for melanoma is generally associated with the worst overall survival due to high rates of early recurrence and disease progression. Across a handful of retrospective studies that focus solely on pulmonary metastasectomy for malignant melanoma, 5-year survival ranges from 20% to 35%.[21,22] Chua and colleagues[22] observed significant rates of progression-free and overall survival with pulmonary metastasectomy, especially in melanoma patients with solitary metastases less than 2 cm in size. After complete resection of pulmonary metastases, median progression-free survival was 10 months and overall 5-year survival was 38%. Metastasis greater than 2 cm in size and a positive surgical margin were independent risk factors for decreased progression-free and overall survival. The presence of more than 1 pulmonary metastatic lesion was also independently associated with decreased survival.

There is limited published evidence regarding pulmonary metastasectomy for melanoma and involvement of intrathoracic lymph nodes. Of 36 patients identified as having intrathoracic nodal metastases (12%), median survival was decreased (16 months with nodal disease vs 27 months without nodal disease).[22] There was a trend toward shorter progression-free and overall survival in patients with lymph node involvement, although this did not reach statistical significance. Lymph node sampling or dissection was not routinely performed and only used in patients with abnormal or bulky lymphadenopathy identified on preoperative imaging or intraoperatively. In contrast, subset analysis of melanoma patients in the IRLM, in which 8% of the patients harbored nodal metastases, there was no apparent impact of nodal status on survival.[23] The investigators acknowledged that patients with clinically positive lymph nodes were likely excluded from metastasectomy and also the number of patients was relatively small. Although it is reasonable to suspect that lymph node involvement is associated with decreased survival, there is no robust evidence to support the viewpoint that surgical resection should be foregone in such patients, especially if no other effective treatment options are available. With the evolution of targeted therapy with BRAF-kinase inhibition for BRAF mutation–positive metastatic melanoma patients, treatment with vemurafenib in combination with surgery for residual disease may become the optimal strategy. Preliminary data indicate that post-resection disease-free survival may be prolonged in such patients.[24]

Head and Neck Squamous Cell Carcinoma

Pulmonary metastases developing in patients with head and neck cancer has generally been associated with poor long-term survival. In spite of the expected poor prognosis, a 5-year survival rate of 30% was observed in a recent meta-analysis of reports concerning pulmonary resection of SCC metastases.[25] Negative prognostic factors included short disease-free interval, male gender, primary tumor in oral cavity, presence of cervical lymph node metastases, and incomplete resection. Although the prognostic relevance of intrathoracic lymph node involvement was not examined in this meta-analysis, Winter and colleagues[26] observed inferior survival in patients with hilar or mediastinal lymph node metastases in patients undergoing metastasectomy. Intraoperative nodal assessment was not routinely performed in this study, and the number of node-positive patients was relatively small (n = 5, 21%). Although the difference in survival was not statistically significant comparing node-positive and node-negative patients, there were no 5-year survivors in the node-positive group.

Breast Carcinoma

The data concerning mediastinal lymph node involvement and pulmonary resection of metastatic breast cancer are sparse. Generally, treatment of metastatic breast cancer consists primarily of chemotherapy, hormonal therapy, or targeted molecular therapy. Pulmonary metastasectomy is occasionally performed to provide tissue for molecular testing and may confer a modest survival benefit in highly selected patients, although cure is typically not expected. In 2 studies concerning pulmonary metastasectomy for breast cancer, nodal metastases were discovered in approximately 30% of patients who underwent lymph node dissection, although the number of node-positive patients was small, and nodal metastasis was not an independent predictor of worse survival.[27,28] Yoshimoto and colleagues[29] observed unexpected hilar or mediastinal lymph node involvement in 44% (n = 37) of patients undergoing systematic hilar and mediastinal lymph node dissection. Although 10-year survival was reduced in node-positive patients

(34% vs 44%), the difference was not statistically significant (*P* = .186).

Incidence and Prognostic Value of Nodal Status by Histology

The predominant theme in the literature is that intrathoracic lymph node involvement in patients with pulmonary metastasis is associated with decreased survival regardless of primary tumor histology. **Table 1** summarizes the results from the published data reviewed above. The precise prognostic value of intrathoracic nodal metastases is uncertain, because the initial report from the IRLM and another more recent and large study of 575 patients undergoing pulmonary metastasectomy[30] failed to identify intrathoracic lymph node involvement as a statistically significant prognostic factor after multivariate analysis. Many of the studies are single-institution retrospective analyses of patients in whom systematic mediastinal lymph node dissection was not routinely performed, so the exact incidence of nodal metastasis is likely underestimated. No randomized controlled data exist confirming long-term survival after pulmonary metastasectomy, much less the effect of concomitant intrathoracic lymph node dissection.

DOES N1 VERSUS N2 LYMPH NODE DISEASE MATTER?

There is no compelling evidence that N2 nodal disease is worse than N1 nodal disease with regard to survival after pulmonary metastasectomy. Pfannschmidt and colleagues[16] offer some insight into whether hilar or mediastinal lymph node involvement makes a difference. In 245 patients with various primary tumor histologies, the rate of intrathoracic lymph node involvement was 33%. Although median survival was significantly decreased in patients with N1 versus N0 and N1 + N2 versus N0 disease, there was no statistically significant difference between patients with N1 versus N2 disease.[16] Although hilar nodal spread was a risk factor for mediastinal involvement, 13 patients had mediastinal nodal disease in the absence of hilar or intrapulmonary nodal disease. Skip nodal metastases were most common in sarcoma patients. Similarly, Renaud and colleagues[3] reported that the presence of N2 disease with colorectal metastases to the lung did not confer further decreased survival, although any nodal disease was associated with a 50% decrease in 5-year survival. Winter and colleagues[11] also observed similar results in RCC patients with pulmonary metastases, in whom the largest decrement in survival occurred with any nodal metastasis, and location of nodal involvement did not seem to have a major effect.

Risk factors for intrathoracic lymph node metastases include increasing number and size of pulmonary metastases, although this has not been a consistent finding across the literature. The biology of intrathoracic nodal disease in the setting of pulmonary metastases is not well understood and may differ from primary lung cancer based on the absence of a clear relationship between size and location of metastatic lesions and lymph node station involved. It remains unclear if intrathoracic lymph node metastases originate from the metastatic lesion itself or from the primary tumor, although both seem possible.

DOES MEDIASTINAL LYMPHADENECTOMY IMPROVE SURVIVAL?

Although current evidence suggests that intrathoracic lymph node status is an important prognostic factor in pulmonary metastasectomy, whether performance of a systematic and complete mediastinal lymphadenectomy improves survival is unanswered at this time. In resection of primary lung cancer, mediastinal lymph node dissection, as opposed to sampling, provides the most

Table 1
Summary of incidence and prognosis of intrathoracic nodal metastases

Primary Tumor Histology	Incidence of Intrathoracic Lymph Node Involvement (%)	5-Year Survival After R0 Resection (%)[31]	Median Survival N− vs N+ (mo)
Colorectal	30	45	94 vs 42[3]
Renal cell	35	40	107 vs 37[13]
Sarcoma	15	40	47 vs 18[17]
Germ cell tumor	25	80	Not reported
Melanoma	10	25	27 vs 16[22]
Head and neck SCC	35	30	29 vs 11[26]
Breast	30	40	85 vs 38[29]

accurate staging, although it does not translate to improved survival.[32] Kudelin and colleagues[33] retrospectively examined 116 RCC patients over an 11-year experience who underwent pulmonary metastasectomy with systematic mediastinal lymph node dissection with curative intent. Complete resection was achieved in 93% of patients, and 35% of patients received systemic therapy prior to surgery. Although patients with intrathoracic lymph node metastases had reduced survival compared with patients without nodal disease, the median survival was reasonable at 37 months and significantly longer than in prior reports.[11,16] The investigators suggested that complete lymphadenectomy in combination with systemic therapy in patients with mediastinal or hilar nodal disease may result in prolonged survival, although the absence of a control group undergoing sampling or no lymph node assessment weakens this assertion. Winter and colleagues,[11] in a multivariate analysis, observed that tumor-infiltrated mediastinal lymph nodes were an independent prognostic factor in metastatic RCC. They performed a matched pair analysis among 110 patients who underwent mediastinal lymph node dissection and 111 patients who did not at metastasectomy and demonstrated a trend toward improved survival in patients who underwent mediastinal lymph node dissection ($P = .068$). Seebacher and colleagues[34] similarly identified a trend toward improved 5-year survival (31% vs 25%) in patients who underwent pulmonary metastasectomy and mediastinal lymph node dissection (n = 158) versus lymph node sampling (n = 112) for various primary tumor histologies, but the difference was not statistically significant. In spite of these suggestive studies, the evidence that lymph node dissection improves survival in patients undergoing pulmonary metastasectomy is lacking.

WHICH PATIENTS SHOULD UNDERGO MEDIASTINAL LYMPH NODE DISSECTION?

Because many thoracic surgeons currently perform mediastinal lymph node dissection or sampling only when suspicious nodes are identified on imaging or intraoperative findings, the evidence for this practice should be re-examined. The sensitivity of CT imaging in detecting intrathoracic lymph node metastases in RCC has been reported to be only 84%.[11] PET-CT is not expected to significantly increase sensitivity in the detection of nodal disease in RCC patients given that FDG avidity is not assured for this particular histology. Moreover, in 63 consecutive patients undergoing pulmonary metastasectomy

and systematic lymph node dissection for multiple tumor types, Loehe and colleagues[35] discovered positive mediastinal lymph nodes in 14% (n = 9) of patients. All of these patients had preoperative CT scans without enlarged mediastinal lymph nodes, and the metastases were unexpected. A more recent and larger study of 209 patients by Seebacher and colleagues[34] observed a rate of unexpected intrathoracic nodal metastases in 17% of patients undergoing pulmonary metastasectomy for diverse histologies. These patients universally underwent CT and PET assessment of mediastinal lymph nodes prior to surgery. The cumulative evidence argues for routine mediastinal lymph node assessment in all patients undergoing pulmonary metastasectomy.

Although the therapeutic effect of routine lymph node dissection or sampling is uncertain, its prognostic importance seems to be clear. As many as 1 in 5 patients undergoing metastasectomy prove to have unexpected nodal metastases and are expected to have inferior survival. Given the progress in systemic therapy, it remains to be seen if protocols will improve survival in these at-risk patients. Additionally, knowledge of mediastinal nodal involvement likely will have an impact on selection of patients for metastasectomy. Although the authors do not support recommendations that nodal metastasis always precludes metastasectomy,[36] it is circumspect to avoid extended resections and pneumonectomy in patients found to harbor nodal metastases. Indications for intrathoracic node assessment during pulmonary metastasectomy include

- FDG-avid or enlarged intrathoracic nodes detected on PET and CT imaging
- Primary tumor histology is colorectal (especially rectal) or RCC
- Further adjuvant therapy would be offered for nodal metastases
- Large solitary metastasis greater than 3 cm or multiple lesions
- Bilobectomy, pneumonectomy, or extended resection required for complete resection

Based on the authors' review, a multicenter randomized trial is conceivable to settle the controversy regarding the role of mediastinal lymph node dissection in pulmonary metastasectomy.

REFERENCES

1. Pastorino U, Buyse M, Friedel G, et al. Long-term results of lung metastasectomy: prognostic analyses based on 5206 cases. J Thorac Cardiovasc Surg 1997;113(1):37–49.

2. Internullo E, Cassivi SD, Van Raemdonck D, et al. Pulmonary metastasectomy: a survey of current practice amongst members of the european society of thoracic surgeons. J Thorac Oncol 2008;3(11):1257–66.

3. Renaud S, Alifano M, Falcoz PE, et al. Does nodal status influence survival? Results of a 19-year systematic lymphadenectomy experience during lung metastasectomy of colorectal cancer. Interact Cardiovasc Thorac Surg 2014;18(4):482–7.

4. Meimarakis G, Spelsberg F, Angele M, et al. Resection of pulmonary metastases from colon and rectal cancer: factors to predict survival differ regarding to the origin of the primary tumor. Ann Surg Oncol 2014;21(8):2563–72.

5. Welter S, Jacobs J, Krbek T, et al. Prognostic impact of lymph node involvement in pulmonary metastases from colorectal cancer. Eur J Cardiothorac Surg 2007;31(2):167–72.

6. Hamaji M, Cassivi SD, Shen KR, et al. Is lymph node dissection required in pulmonary metastasectomy for colorectal adenocarcinoma? Ann Thorac Surg 2012;94(6):1796–800.

7. Riquet M, Foucault C, Cazes A, et al. Pulmonary resection for metastases of colorectal adenocarcinoma. Ann Thorac Surg 2010;89(2):375–80.

8. Renaud S, Falcoz PE, Olland A, et al. The intrathoracic lymph node ratio seems to be a better prognostic factor than the level of lymph node involvement in lung metastasectomy of colorectal carcinoma. Interact Cardiovasc Thorac Surg 2015;20(2):215–21.

9. Bolukbas S, Sponholz S, Kudelin N, et al. Risk factors for lymph node metastases and prognosticators of survival in patients undergoing pulmonary metastasectomy for colorectal cancer. Ann Thorac Surg 2014;97(6):1926–32.

10. Renaud S, Falcoz PE, Olland A, et al. Should mediastinal lymphadenectomy be performed during lung metastasectomy of renal cell carcinoma? Interact Cardiovasc Thorac Surg 2013;16(4):525–8.

11. Winter H, Meimarakis G, Angele MK, et al. Tumor infiltrated hilar and mediastinal lymph nodes are an independent prognostic factor for decreased survival after pulmonary metastasectomy in patients with renal cell carcinoma. J Urol 2010;184(5):1888–94.

12. Meimarakis G, Angele M, Staehler M, et al. Evaluation of a new prognostic score (munich score) to predict long-term survival after resection of pulmonary renal cell carcinoma metastases. Am J Surg 2011;202(2):158–67.

13. Renaud S, Falcoz PE, Alifano M, et al. Systematic lymph node dissection in lung metastasectomy of renal cell carcinoma: An 18 years of experience. J Surg Oncol 2014;109(8):823–9.

14. Smith R, Demmy TL. Pulmonary metastasectomy for soft tissue sarcoma. Surg Oncol Clin N Am 2012;21(2):269–86.

15. Kon Z, Martin L. Resection for thoracic metastases from sarcoma. Oncology (Williston Park) 2011;25(12):1198–204.

16. Pfannschmidt J, Klode J, Muley T, et al. Nodal involvement at the time of pulmonary metastasectomy: Experiences in 245 patients. Ann Thorac Surg 2006;81(2):448–54.

17. Pfannschmidt J, Klode J, Muley T, et al. Pulmonary metastasectomy in patients with soft tissue sarcomas: Experiences in 50 patients. J Thorac Cardiovasc Surg 2006;54(7):489–92.

18. Pfannschmidt J, Hoffmann H, Dienemann H. Thoracic metastasectomy for nonseminomatous germ cell tumors. J Thorac Oncol 2010;5:S182–6.

19. Pfannschmidt J, Zabeck H, Muley T, et al. Pulmonary metastasectomy following chemotherapy in patients with testicular tumors: Experience in 52 patients. Thorac Cardiovasc Surg 2006;54(7):484–8.

20. Kesler KA, Kruter LE, Perkins SM, et al. Survival after resection for metastatic testicular nonseminomatous germ cell cancer to the lung or mediastinum. Ann Thorac Surg 2011;91(4):1085–93 [discussion: 1093].

21. Petersen RP, Hanish SI, Haney JC, et al. Improved survival with pulmonary metastasectomy: an analysis of 1720 patients with pulmonary metastatic melanoma. J Thorac Cardiovasc Surg 2007;133(1):104–10.

22. Chua TC, Scolyer RA, Kennedy CW, et al. Surgical management of melanoma lung metastasis: An analysis of survival outcomes in 292 consecutive patients. Ann Surg Oncol 2012;19(6):1774–81.

23. Leo F, Cagini L, Rocmans P, et al. Lung metastases from melanoma: when is surgical treatment warranted? Br J Cancer 2000;83(5):569–72.

24. He M, Lovell J, Ng BL, et al. Post-operative survival following metastasectomy for patients receiving braf inhibitor therapy is associated with duration of pre-operative treatment and elective indication. J Surg Oncol 2015;111(8):980–4.

25. Young ER, Diakos E, Khalid-Raja M, et al. Resection of subsequent pulmonary metastases from treated head and neck squamous cell carcinoma: Systematic review and meta-analysis. Clin Otolaryngol 2015;40(3):208–18.

26. Winter H, Meimarakis G, Hoffmann G, et al. Does surgical resection of pulmonary metastases of head and neck cancer improve survival? Ann Surg Oncol 2008;15(10):2915–26.

27. Meimarakis G, Ruttinger D, Stemmler J, et al. Prolonged overall survival after pulmonary metastasectomy in patients with breast cancer. Ann Thorac Surg 2013;95(4):1170–80.

28. Welter S, Jacobs J, Krbek T, et al. Pulmonary metastases of breast cancer. When is resection indicated? Eur J Cardiothorac Surg 2008;34(6):1228–34.

29. Yoshimoto M, Tada K, Nishimura S, et al. Favourable long-term results after surgical removal of lung metastases of breast cancer. Breast Cancer Res Treat 2008;110(3):485–91.

30. Casiraghi M, De Pas T, Maisonneuve P, et al. A 10-year single-center experience on 708 lung metastasectomies: The evidence of the "international registry of lung metastases". J Thorac Oncol 2011;6(8):1373–8.

31. Kaifi JT, Gusani NJ, Deshaies I, et al. Indications and approach to surgical resection of lung metastases. J Surg Oncol 2010;102(2):187–95.

32. Darling GE, Allen MS, Decker PA, et al. Randomized trial of mediastinal lymph node sampling versus complete lymphadenectomy during pulmonary resection in the patient with n0 or n1 (less than hilar) non-small cell carcinoma: Results of the american college of surgery oncology group z0030 trial. J Thorac Cardiovasc Surg 2011; 141(3):662–70.

33. Kudelin N, Bolukbas S, Eberlein M, et al. Metastasectomy with standardized lymph node dissection for metastatic renal cell carcinoma: An 11-year single-center experience. Ann Thorac Surg 2013; 96(1):265–70.

34. Seebacher G, Decker S, Fischer JR, et al. Unexpected lymph node disease in resections for pulmonary metastases. Ann Thorac Surg 2015; 99(1):231–6.

35. Loehe F, Kobinger S, Hatz RA, et al. Value of systematic mediastinal lymph node dissection during pulmonary metastasectomy. Ann Thorac Surg 2001;72(1):225–9.

36. Garcia-Yuste M, Cassivi S, Paleru C. Thoracic lymphatic involvement in patients having pulmonary metastasectomy incidence and the effect on prognosis. J Thorac Oncol 2010;5(6):S166–9.

Induction Therapy for Thymoma

Usman Ahmad, MD[a],*, James Huang, MD[b]

KEYWORDS

- Thymic tumors • Induction treatment • Neoadjuvant • Chemotherapy • Chemoradiation

KEY POINTS

- Although surgery is the mainstay of treatment of most thymic tumors, they are also chemosensitive and radiosensitive.
- Locally advanced thymic tumors may pose challenges to complete resection given the anatomic confines of the mediastinum.
- Induction therapy with chemotherapy or radiation therapy prior to surgery may improve surgical resectability.
- Although response to induction chemotherapy or chemoradiotherapy seems comparable, greater tumor necrosis has been observed after chemoradiotherapy, albeit at a potential cost of higher toxicity.

INTRODUCTION

Thymic neoplasms are rare malignancies with an incidence of approximately 2.2 to 2.6/million/y for thymomas and even less for thymic carcinomas (0.3–0.6/million/y).[1] They represent, however, the most common tumors of the mediastinum encountered by thoracic surgeons, and a notable proportion of these tumors present at an advanced stage. Local invasion into surrounding mediastinal structures (Masaoka-Koga stage III)[2] or intrathoracic metastases to the pleura or pericardium (stage IVA) can pose a challenge to complete resection. In a worldwide data set of 4987 cases assembled by the International Thymic Malignancy Interest Group,[3] approximately 30% of the tumors were Masaoka-Koga stages III and IVA, and 11% of the tumors reported by the Japanese Association for Research on the Thymus were stage III thymomas.[4]

The stage of the tumor and completeness of resection have been consistently found the most significant prognostic factors.[5] Early-stage, localized tumors (Masaoka-Koga stages I and II) are typically treated with surgical resection alone, with prolonged survival outcomes and 10-year overall survival rates of 80% to 90%.[6] The poorer outcomes historically associated with locally advanced stage thymic tumors have led clinicians to use multimodality strategies with the addition of chemotherapy and radiotherapy to surgery.

GENERAL APPROACH TO THE TREATMENT OF LOCALLY ADVANCED THYMIC TUMORS

Thymic tumors are generally considered a surgical disease and a complete resection is the primary goal. Successful treatment of locally advanced tumors requires careful selection of patients and surgical approach and consideration of neoadjuvant therapies that may improve the likelihood of a complete resection.

Disclosures: None.

[a] Division of Thoracic Surgery, Department of Cardiothoracic Surgery, Heart and Vascular Institute, Cleveland Clinic, 9500 Euclid Avenue, J4-1, Cleveland, OH 44195, USA; [b] Thoracic Service, Department of Surgery, Memorial Sloan Kettering Cancer Center, 1275 York Avenue, New York, NY 10065, USA
* Corresponding author.
E-mail address: ahmadu@ccf.org

The general approach to patients with locally advanced thymic tumors should involve a multidisciplinary evaluation, including the thoracic surgeon, medical oncologist, radiation oncologist, radiologist, pathologist, and neurologist (for patients with concomitant myasthenia gravis). Discussion of the treatment plan in the setting of a multidisciplinary tumor board can greatly facilitate the coordination of care for these challenging cases.

Radiographic evaluation with a high-resolution CT scan with intravenous contrast (preferentially given through the left or right upper extremity to opacify the innominate vein or right brachiocephalic vein if there is concern for invasion of these structures) is essential for delineating the anatomic relationships of the tumor and adjacent organs.[7] The value of PET scanning in these patients remains unclear but may be more helpful in patients with thymic carcinomas to evaluate the extent of disease, given their more aggressive nature and higher propensity towards distant metastasis.[8]

If preoperative therapy is planned, tissue diagnosis is needed before initiating induction treatment. This can generally be obtained through needle biopsy, preferentially a core biopsy.[9] The risk of seeding by the needle is extremely low and certainly no higher than attempts at biopsy via mediastinotomy (Chamberlain procedure) or by thoracoscopy, where cells can be shed into the open pleural space in the course of biopsying the mass. After completion of induction therapy, the patient is restaged with another contrast CT scan to evaluate response to treatment and extent of disease.

INDUCTION CHEMOTHERAPY IN THYMOMA

Thymomas are considered chemosensitive tumors and a variety of combinations of chemotherapy regimens have been reported with varying response rates.[5] The sensitivity of thymomas to chemotherapy was well established by 2 cooperative group trials, 1 examining the cisplatin, doxorubicin, cyclophosphamide (CAP) regimen led by Eastern Cooperative Oncology Group[10] and 1 examining etoposide-cisplatin (EP) led by the European Organisation for Research and Treatment of Cancer[11] in patients with metastatic or unresectable disease. Response rates were notable and comparable with acceptable toxicity across both regimens.[10,11]

In general, the literature on induction therapy is comprised largely of small retrospective case series, but these collectively suggest that combination regimens are well tolerated and a majority of the patients in the reported studies were able to proceed to resection with promising resection rates (**Table 1**). In these studies thymomas have demonstrated marked chemosensitivity with clinical response rates of approximately 62% to 100% and complete resection rates of 22% to 92%.

Unsurprisingly there are no randomized controlled trials on induction therapy in this rare disease, but a few prospective single-arm trials have been conducted and are worth noting. The CAP regimen was used as induction therapy in patients with unresectable thymoma in a single-arm prospective trial published by Kim and colleagues,[12] which included 22 patients with locally advanced disease. Patients received neoadjuvant chemotherapy with CAP and prednisone, followed by resection, postoperative radiotherapy (PORT), and consolidation chemotherapy; 17 patients had some radiographic response and 6 of 16 patients had greater than 80% tumor necrosis on pathologic evaluation. At 5 years, disease-free survival was 77% and overall survival was 95%.

In a phase II study conducted by the Japan Clinical Oncology Group, either dose-dense chemotherapy (cisplatin, vincristine, doxorubicin, and etoposide) or radiation was administered followed by resection. Resectable patients underwent surgery and PORT whereas unresectable patients received radiation only. In the chemotherapy group, 62% of patients had radiographic response and 14% had complete pathologic response.[13]

Lucchi and colleagues[14] reported a prospective analysis of 30 stages III and IVA thymoma patients who underwent induction with cisplatin, epirubicin, and etoposide. They noted 73% response rate and 77% complete resection rate.

More recently multi-institutional collaborations have led to large retrospective database analyses. In a recent report from the Japanese Association for Research of the Thymus, 441 patients with clinical stage III thymoma were evaluated. Among those, 113 received induction treatment. Induction treatment response was 52%; however, induction was associated with worse prognosis. The investigators concluded that this is likely because patients with more advanced disease received induction treatment.[4]

In a report from the European Society of Thoracic Surgeons database,[15] 370 stage III thymoma patients were reported. Induction and adjuvant treatments were administered at the discretion of the multidisciplinary team. Induction was generally administered, however, to patients deemed to have unresectable disease. Most common chemotherapy regimen was cisplatin,

Table 1
Results of multimodality treatment in thymoma using induction chemotherapy

Author	y	N	Stage	Chemotherapy	Response Rate (%)	Complete Resection Rate (%)	Postoperative Radiotherapy	Disease-free Survival	Overall Survival
Prospective									
Macchiarini et al,[37]	1988–1990	7	III	Cisplatin, epirubicin, etoposide	100	57	45 Gy (R0)	—	—
Rea et al,[38]	1985–1991	16	III, IVA	Doxorubicin, cisplatin, vincristine, cyclophosphamide	100	69	11 cases	—	70%—3 y
Berruti et al,[39]	1990–1992	6	III, IVA	Doxorubicin, cisplatin, vincristine, cyclophosphamide	83	83	—	—	—
Venuta et al,[40]	1989–onwards	15	III	Cisplatin, epirubicin, etoposide	67	91	40 Gy (R0)	—	—
Kim et al,[12]	1990–2000	22	III, IVA	Cisplatin, doxorubicin, cyclophosphamide, prednisone	77	76	50 Gy (R0)	77%—5 y	95%—5 y
Yokoi et al,[41]	1988–2003	14	III, IVA	Cisplatin, doxorubicin, methylprednisolone	93	22	50 Gy	—	89%—5 y and 10 y
Lucchi et al,[14]	1989–2004	30	III, IVA	Cisplatin, epirubicin, etoposide	73	77	45 Gy (R0)	—	82%—10 y
Kunitoh et al,[13]	1997–2005	21	III	Cisplatin, vincristine, doxorubicin, etoposide	62	43	48 Gy (R0)	32–8 y	69%—8 y
Retrospective									
Bretti et al,[42]	1990–1992	25	III, IVA	Doxorubicin, cisplatin, vincristine, cyclophosphamide (18 cases) Cisplatin, etoposide (7 cases)	72	44	45 Gy (R0)	—	—
Yamada et al,[4]	1991–2010	113	III	Not specified	52	—	—	—	—
Leuzzi et al,[15]	1990–2010	88	III	Cisplatin, doxorubicin, cyclophosphamide, vincristine	—	65	—	—	—

doxorubicin, cyclophosphamide, and vincristine. Induction therapy was administered to 88 (25%) of the patients. No association between induction treatment and cancer-specific or recurrence-free survival was noted. The induction group, however, consisted of patients with more advanced disease and the investigators were unable to draw firm conclusions about the benefit of induction therapy in their data set.

Collectively these studies suggest that induction chemotherapy is feasible and well tolerated with an acceptable toxicity profile and results in substantial response rates in locally advanced tumors.

INDUCTION CHEMORADIATION IN THYMOMA

The addition of radiation to induction chemotherapy has been used in locally advanced malignancies when there are concerns about the ability to obtain an R0 resection (superior sulcus lung cancer or esophageal cancer)[16,17] and this strategy has also been examined in thymic tumors.

The efficacy of chemoradiation in thymic malignancies was established by a prospective multi-institutional cooperative group trial led by Loehrer and colleagues.[18] Patients with localized unresectable thymoma and thymic carcinoma underwent 4 cycles of cisplatin, doxorubicin, and cyclophosphamide followed by 54 Gy of radiation as definitive therapy. Among the 23 assessable patients, the overall response rate to initial chemotherapy was 69.6%. After radiation, 1 patient with partial response had complete response. Four patients who previously had minimal response now showed complete or partial response. No patient had progression during radiation. The 5-year overall survival was 53%.

The use of chemoradiation as an induction strategy was described by Wright and colleagues,[19] who reported a series of 10 patients at the Massachusetts General Hospital with stages III and IVA thymic tumors, using induction treatment consisting of cisplatin and etoposide with concurrent radiation dose of 40 Gy to 45 Gy. Four patients had partial response; however, 8 patients had an R0 resection whereas 2 had an R1 resection. Four patients had a pathologic complete response. The opportunity to achieve pathologic complete responses with concurrent chemoradiation has led to interest in pursuing this as a strategy in patients thought unresectable or questionably resectable.

The encouraging response to induction chemoradiation noted in the studies (discussed previously) led to a multi-institutional phase II study of induction treatment with cisplatin, etoposide, and 45 Gy of radiation.[20] During the 5-year study period, 22 patients with stage III disease were enrolled at 4 institutions. Specific inclusion criteria included tumor diameter greater than 8 cm, tumor diameter 5 cm to 8 cm with irregular borders/heterogeneous appearance/ectopic calcification, or vascular invasion. There were 7 thymic carcinoma and 14 thymoma patients; 21 completed induction treatment and a partial radiographic response was noted in 10 (47%) patients. Grade 3 or 4 toxicity was noted in 9 cases (41%). All 21 patients were surgically explored, 17 (77%) underwent an R0 resection, 3 (14%) had an R1, and 1 (5%) had R2 resection. No patient had a complete pathologic response; however, in 5 cases, less than 10% viable tumor was noted. Postoperative complications were noted in 8 (36%) patients. Two patients died in the perioperative period and 1 had undergone a pneumonectomy and succumbed to respiratory failure from aspiration, whereas the other had an R2 resection due to aortic involvement and had an intraoperative cardiac arrest with subsequent multiorgan failure. At 5 years, the freedom from progression was 83% and overall survival was 71% for the overall cohort of 22 patients.

Other findings that are of interest for future studies include the correlation of high maximum standard uptake value with more aggressive histology. In addition, thymic carcinomas seemed to have a greater response to induction chemoradiation compared with thymomas, because 4 of 5 tumors with less than 10% viable tumor were thymic carcinomas.[20]

The studies reporting the use of induction chemoradiation seem to have at least comparable radiographic response rates to induction chemotherapy alone and potentially higher pathologic response rates (**Table 2**). A note of caution is in order, however, because the issue of toxicity must be considered. Although induction chemoradiation has been routinely and safely used in esophageal cancer and for superior sulcus tumors, the general treatment volume is small. Thymomas, on the other hand, can be sizable, with a corresponding radiation field that is large and centered over the mediastinum, which may lead to greater toxicity before surgery as well as a greater risk of perioperative complications.[19–21] Serious adverse events occurred in more than 40% of patients in the phase II trial of EP/45 Gy, and perioperative mortality was 9%.[20] Furthermore long-term toxicities from radiotherapy, especially the risk of coronary and valvular disease given the location of the treatment field, must also be taken into account, which may compound the cardiotoxicity from doxorubicin. The risk of subsequent radiation-induced malignancy also must be considered. No data yet exist to determine whether a higher

Table 2
Results of multimodality treatment in thymoma using induction chemoradiation therapy

Author	y	N	Stage	Chemotherapy	Radiation	Response Rate	Complete Resection	Disease-Free Survival	Overall Survival
Prospective									
Loehrer et al,[18,a]	1983–1995	23	III, IV	Cisplatin, cyclophosphamide, doxorubicin	54 Gy	70	No resection	—	53%—5 y
Korst et al,[20]	2007–2012	21	I, II, III	Cisplatin, etoposide	45 Gy	47	77	83%—5 y (freedom from progression)	71%—5 y
Retrospective									
Wright et al,[19]	1997–2006	10	III, IVA	Cisplatin, etoposide	40–45 Gy	40	80	—	69%—5 y

[a] Chemoradiation as definitive therapy only. No surgery.

pathologic response rate with the addition of radiation to induction chemotherapy bears out with a long-term survival benefit or is offset potentially by higher toxicity.

INDUCTION RADIATION IN THYMOMA

The role of induction radiation only has been reported in a few small retrospective series and variable outcomes are noted.

In a series of 34 stage III thymoma patients, 8 received preoperative radiation with cobalt 60 whereas 26 did not. Patients who underwent a complete resection had improved survival; however, there was no difference in overall survival between patients who did or did not receive preoperative radiation.[22] More modern radiation treatments have since been reported by others. Ribet and colleagues[23] reported a series of 113 patients where 19 patients had preoperative radiation. In this group, complete resection was achieved in 10 of 19 patients. The overall 5-year survival in these 19 patients was 44%. Akaogi and colleagues[24] reported a series of 12 patients with thymic tumor invading the great vessels (vena cava, pulmonary artery, and aorta). Patients were treated with preoperative radiation (12–21 Gy). On exploration, 1 patient had stage IVA disease. The rate of complete resection was 75%. Ten patients also received adjuvant radiation (mean, 42.3 Gy). The overall survival was 72% at 5 years and 48% at 10 years.

Most institutions now favor the use of chemotherapy in the induction setting. In a multi-institutional study from European Society of Thoracic Surgeons database, only 12 of 2030 (1%) of patients underwent induction radiation alone.[25] A review of the International Thymic Malignancy Interest Group database showed that for thymic carcinomas, 48 of 1042 (6%) of the cases had induction radiation only.[26]

SPECIAL CONSIDERATIONS WITH STAGE IVA DISEASE

In extensive pleural disease, extrapleural pneumonectomy can potentially achieve a macroscopic complete resection and has been shown feasible. An additional potential benefit is the ability to provide hemithoracic radiation without the risk of pneumonitis. In patients with limited pleural disease, partial pleurectomy is undertaken. In both scenarios, induction treatment is usually chemotherapy only, given the size of the necessary treatment field. To improve pleural disease control, other modalities have been explored.

In a series of 35 stage IVA patients with thymoma (17), thymic carcinoma (4), and recurrent thymoma (14), induction chemotherapy was administered to all thymic carcinoma and 13 thymoma patients. One patient underwent EPP, whereas the remaining underwent local resection of involved areas. The pleural space was intraoperatively perfused with cisplatin and doxorubicin at 45°C for 60 minutes; 90-day mortality was 2.5%. Local control was not achieved in thymic carcinoma patients and all died within 4 years. After median follow-up of 62 months, the 5-year and 10-year progression-free survival rates were 61% and 43%, respectively, for primary thymomas, and 48% and 18%, respectively, for recurrent thymomas.[27] Lang-Lazdunski and colleagues[28] popularized the use of pleural lavage with povidine-iodine solution. In a series of 6 thymoma patients with pleural disease, induction chemotherapy was administered followed by complete pleurectomy. Povidine-iodine solution (diluted in a 1:10 ratio in sterile water and heated to 40°C–41°C) was instilled in the pleural space for at least 15 minutes. There were no in-hospital deaths. After median follow-up of 18 months, 1 patient had died of unrelated reasons and 1 patient underwent reresection for recurrence whereas the remaining 4 patients had no evidence of disease.

These treatment protocols may have utility in the treatment of pleural disease where the major concern is the difficulty of surgery to truly achieve an R0 resection in the setting of extensive pleural metastasis. To date, however, there are no validated prospective data yet that demonstrate efficacy in these difficult cases.

ROLE OF TARGETED THERAPIES

Thymic tumors have been noted to harbor several mutations that are associated with prognostication or with targetable pathways.[29,30] Despite several phase I studies in unresectable patients, no significant and consistent response has been shown.

Epidermal growth factor receptor was noted to be overexpressed in 70% of thymomas and 50% of thymic carcinomas; however, activating mutations are rarely seen.[29] Two phase II studies using gefitinib and erlotinib showed poor response rates in chemorefractory patients.[31,32] Similarly, KIT overexpression has reported in thymic carcinomas; however, less than 10% of the tumors harbor a KIT mutation and to date no response has been reported with the use of imatinib.[33]

More recently, insulinlike growth factor receptor overexpression has been shown in thymic tumors[34] and a phase II study is under way.[35]

Partial responses to cetuximab have been reported and a phase II study of cetuximab in chemorefractory advanced thymic tumors showed partial response in 5 of 49 patients.[36] Given these responses, a phase II study of CAP plus cetuximab as induction therapy followed by surgery in locally advanced chemo-naïve patients was designed and is currently ongoing at the Memorial Sloan Kettering Cancer Center (NCT01025089). Patients receive 4 cycles of CAP concurrently with cetuximab on a weekly basis, followed by surgical resection. The recent developments with immunotherapy have raised the potential for opportunities to investigate novel combined therapy approaches in these tumors, but to date there is no targeted therapy that is in routine clinical use in the induction setting outside of the aforementioned clinical trial.

WHAT IS THE ACTUAL BENEFIT OF INDUCTION THERAPY?

Complete surgical resection is the cornerstone in management of resectable thymic tumors. Other than tumor stage, an R0 resection has been the most consistent prognostic factor noted in retrospective and prospective studies. Therefore, any treatment that can improve the rate of R0 resection may have an impact on the long-term outcome. There is significant variability among the reported studies; therefore, a direct comparison of rate of complete resection with or without induction treatment is difficult. Promising clinical response and complete resection rates have been reported, however, with the use of induction treatment, making the case for its use in advanced thymic tumors. Continued investigation and, importantly, more accurate and systematic capture of data and outcomes will lead to further refinements in understanding of the optimal treatment strategies for these challenging patients.

REFERENCES

1. de Jong WK, Blaauwgeers JL, Schaapveld M, et al. Thymic epithelial tumours: a population-based study of the incidence, diagnostic procedures and therapy. Eur J Cancer 2008;44:123–30.
2. Koga K, Matsuno Y, Noguchi M, et al. A review of 79 thymomas: modification of staging system and reappraisal of conventional division into invasive and non-invasive thymoma. Pathol Int 1994;44: 359–67.
3. Huang J, Ahmad U, Antonicelli A, et al, International Thymic Malignancy Interest Group International Database Committee and Contributors. Development of the international thymic malignancy interest group international database: an unprecedented resource for the study of a rare group of tumors. J Thorac Oncol 2014;9:1573–8.
4. Yamada Y, Yoshino I, Nakajima J, et al, Japanese Association for Research of the Thymus. Surgical outcomes of patients with stage III thymoma in the Japanese nationwide database. Ann Thorac Surg 2015;100:961–7.
5. Detterbeck FC, Parsons AM. Thymic tumors. Ann Thorac Surg 2004;77:1860–9.
6. Detterbeck FC, Parsons AM. Management of stage I and II thymoma. Thorac Surg Clin 2011;21:59–67.
7. Marom EM, Rosado-de-Christenson ML, Bruzzi JF, et al. Standard report terms for chest computed tomography reports of anterior mediastinal masses suspicious for thymoma. J Thorac Oncol 2011;6: S1717–23.
8. Benveniste MF, Moran CA, Mawlawi O, et al. FDG PET-CT aids in the preoperative assessment of patients with newly diagnosed thymic epithelial malignancies. J Thorac Oncol 2013;8:502–10.
9. Marchevsky A, Marx A, Ströbel P, et al. Policies and reporting guidelines for small biopsy specimens of mediastinal masses. J Thorac Oncol 2011;6: S1724–9.
10. Loehrer PJ Sr, Kim K, Aisner SC, et al. Cisplatin plus doxorubicin plus cyclophosphamide in metastatic or recurrent thymoma: final results of an intergroup trial. The Eastern Cooperative Oncology Group, Southwest Oncology Group, and Southeastern Cancer Study Group. J Clin Oncol 1994;12:1164–8.
11. Giaccone G, Ardizzoni A, Kirkpatrick A, et al. Cisplatin and etoposide combination chemotherapy for locally advanced or metastatic thymoma. A phase II study of the European Organization for Research and Treatment of Cancer Lung Cancer Cooperative Group. J Clin Oncol 1996;14:814–20.
12. Kim ES, Putnam JB, Komaki R, et al. Phase II study of a multidisciplinary approach with induction chemotherapy, followed by surgical resection, radiation therapy, and consolidation chemotherapy for unresectable malignant thymomas: final report. Lung Cancer 2004;44:369–79.
13. Kunitoh H, Tamura T, Shibata T, et al, JCOG Lung Cancer Study Group. A phase II trial of dose-dense chemotherapy, followed by surgical resection and/or thoracic radiotherapy, in locally advanced thymoma: report of a Japan Clinical Oncology Group trial (JCOG 9606). Br J Cancer 2010;103: 6–11.
14. Lucchi M, Melfi F, Dini P, et al. Neoadjuvant chemotherapy for stage III and IVA thymomas: a single-institution experience with a long follow-up. J Thorac Oncol 2006;1:308–13.
15. Leuzzi G, Rocco G, Ruffini E, et al, ESTS Thymic Working Group. Multimodality therapy for locally advanced thymomas: a propensity score-matched

cohort study from the European Society of Thoracic Surgeons Database. J Thorac Cardiovasc Surg 2016;151:47–57.

16. Rusch VW, Giroux DJ, Kraut MJ, et al. Induction chemoradiation and surgical resection for superior sulcus non-small-cell lung carcinomas: long-term results of Southwest Oncology Group Trial 9416 (Intergroup Trial 0160). J Clin Oncol 2007;25:313–8.

17. van Hagen P, Hulshof MC, van Lanschot JJ, et al, CROSS Group. Preoperative chemoradiotherapy for esophageal or junctional cancer. N Engl J Med 2012;366:2074–84.

18. Loehrer PJ Sr, Chen M, Kim K, et al. Cisplatin, doxorubicin, and cyclophosphamide plus thoracic radiation therapy for limited-stage unresectable thymoma: an intergroup trial. J Clin Oncol 1997;15: 3093–9.

19. Wright CD, Choi NC, Wain JC, et al. Induction chemoradiotherapy followed by resection for locally advanced Masaoka stage III and IVA thymic tumors. Ann Thorac Surg 2008;85:385–9.

20. Korst RJ, Bezjak A, Blackmon S, et al. Neoadjuvant chemoradiotherapy for locally advanced thymic tumors: a phase II, multi-institutional clinical trial. J Thorac Cardiovasc Surg 2014;147:36–44.

21. Huang J, Riely GJ, Rosenzweig KE, et al. Multimodality therapy for locally advanced thymomas: state of the art or investigational therapy? Ann Thorac Surg 2008;85:365–7.

22. Yagi K, Hirata T, Fukuse T, et al. Surgical treatment for invasive thymoma, especially when the superior vena cava is invaded. Ann Thorac Surg 1996;61: 521–4.

23. Ribet M, Voisin C, Gosselin B, et al. Lympho-epithelial thymoma. Anatomo-clinical and therapeutic study of 113 cases. Rev Mal Respir 1988;5:53–60 [in French].

24. Akaogi E, Ohara K, Mitsui K, et al. Preoperative radiotherapy and surgery for advanced thymoma with invasion to the great vessels. J Surg Oncol 1996;63:17–22.

25. Ruffini E, Detterbeck F, Van Raemdonck D, et al, European Association of Thoracic Surgeons (ESTS) Thymic Working Group. Tumours of the thymus: a cohort study of prognostic factors from the European Society of Thoracic Surgeons database. Eur J Cardiothorac Surg 2014;46:361–8.

26. Ahmad U, Yao X, Detterbeck F, et al. Thymic carcinoma outcomes and prognosis: results of an international analysis. J Thorac Cardiovasc Surg 2015;149: 95–100.

27. Yellin A, Simansky DA, Ben-Avi R, et al. Resection and heated pleural chemoperfusion in patients with thymic epithelial malignant disease and pleural spread: a single-institution experience. J Thorac Cardiovasc Surg 2013;145:83–7.

28. Belcher E, Hardwick T, Lal R, et al. Induction chemotherapy, cytoreductive surgery and intraoperative hyperthermic pleural irrigation in patients with stage IVA thymoma. Interact Cardiovasc Thorac Surg 2011;12:744–7.

29. Henley JD, Koukoulis GK, Loehrer PJ. Epidermal growth factor receptor expression in invasive thymoma. J Cancer Res Clin Oncol 2002;128:167–70.

30. Girard N, Shen R, Guo T, et al. Comprehensive genomic analysis reveals clinically relevant molecular distinctions between thymic carcinomas and thymomas. Clin Cancer Res 2009;15:6790–9.

31. Kurup A, Burns M, Dropcho S, et al. Phase II study of gefitinib treatment in advanced thymic malignancies. J Clin Oncol 2005;23:381s.

32. Bedano PM, Perkins S, Burns M, et al. A phase II trial of erlotinib plus bevacizumab in patients with recurrent thymoma or thymic carcinoma. J Clin Oncol 2008;26(Suppl):19087.

33. Giaccone G, Rajan A, Ruijter R, et al. Imatinib mesylate in patients with WHO B3 thymomas and thymic carcinomas. J Thorac Oncol 2009;4:1270–3.

34. Girard N, Teruya-Feldstein J, Payabyab EC, et al. Insulin-like growth factor-1 receptor expression in thymic malignancies. J Thorac Oncol 2010;5: 1439–46.

35. Giaccone G. Multicenter phase II study of IMC-A12 in patients with thymoma and thymic carcinoma who have been previously treated with chemotherapy. NCT00965250. Available at: https://clinicaltrials.gov.

36. Rajan A, Carter CA, Berman A, et al. Cixutumumab for patients with recurrent or refractory advanced thymic epithelial tumours: a multicentre, open-label, phase 2 trial. Lancet Oncol 2014;15:191–200.

37. Macchiarini P, Chella A, Ducci F, et al. Neoadjuvant chemotherapy, surgery, and postoperative radiation therapy for invasive thymoma. Cancer 1991;68: 706–13.

38. Rea F, Sartori F, Loy M, et al. Chemotherapy and operation for invasive thymoma. J Thorac Cardiovasc Surg 1993;106:543–9.

39. Berruti A, Borasio P, Roncari A, et al. Neoadjuvant chemotherapy with adriamycin, cisplatin, vincristine and cyclophosphamide (ADOC) in invasive thymomas: results in six patients. Ann Oncol 1993;4: 429–31.

40. Venuta F, Rendina EA, Pescarmona EO, et al. Multimodality treatment of thymoma: a prospective study. Ann Thorac Surg 1997;64:1585–91.

41. Yokoi K, Matsuguma H, Nakahara R, et al. Multidisciplinary treatment for advanced invasive thymoma with cisplatin, doxorubicin, and methylprednisolone. J Thorac Oncol 2007;2:73–8.

42. Bretti S, Berruti A, Loddo C, et al, Piemonte Oncology Network. Multimodal management of stages III-IVa malignant thymoma. Lung Cancer 2004;44:69–77.

Best Approach and Benefit of Plication for Paralyzed Diaphragm

 CrossMark

Eitan Podgaetz, MD, MPH*, Rafael Garza-Castillon Jr, MD,
Rafael S. Andrade, MD

KEYWORDS

- Diaphragm plication • Paralysis • Eventration • Laparoscopy • Thoracoscopy

KEY POINTS

- Diaphragmatic plication is a safe procedure and should be performed for patients with symptomatic diaphragmatic paralysis or eventration.
- The diagnosis of symptomatic diaphragmatic paralysis or eventration is mostly clinical.
- Preoperatively, all patients should have a chest radiograph, pulmonary function tests, and a respiratory quality-of-life questionnaire.
- Although pulmonary function tests are often abnormal in symptomatic patients, these changes are inconsistent and do not correlate with the severity of dyspnea.
- Surgical approaches for plication include open transthoracic, thoracoscopic (with and without mini-thoracotomy), robotic assisted (abdominal or thoracic), open transabdominal, and laparoscopic.

INTRODUCTION
Diaphragmatic Eventration and Diaphragmatic Paralysis

Diaphragmatic eventration is defined as thinning of the diaphragm secondary to a congenital deficiency in its muscular structure; the normal attachments to the sternum, ribs, and dorsolumbar spine are maintained.[1] It is postulated that it occurs embryologically secondary to an abnormal migration of myoblasts from the upper cervical somites into 22 of the 4 embryologic structures that contribute to diaphragm development: the septum transversum (beginning at 4 weeks of gestation) and the pleuroperitoneal membrane (at 8–12 weeks of gestation).[2,3] Clinically, diaphragmatic eventration can be impossible to differentiate from acquired paralysis. Diaphragmatic eventration is rare (incidence <0.05%), more common in male individuals, and more often affects the left hemidiaphragm.[4–6] Most adult patients who have diaphragmatic eventration are asymptomatic and generally present with an elevated hemidiaphragm discovered incidentally on a chest radiograph.[4,7] Symptomatic patients who have diaphragmatic eventration usually present until adulthood because of weight gain or change in lung or chest-wall compliance.[7]

In contrast to true diaphragmatic eventration, diaphragmatic paresis or paralysis is a more common acquired condition. In adults, this condition arises more frequently on the left side. It can result from a number of abnormalities that affect the neuromuscular axis between the cervical spinal cord and the diaphragm.[8] Common causes are idiopathic, iatrogenic phrenic nerve trauma from surgery (eg, cardiac, noncardiac thoracic, and cervical surgeries), tumor invasion of the phrenic nerve (eg, lung and mediastinal tumors), trauma, and rarely, infectious processes.[8–14]

Section of Thoracic and Foregut Surgery, Division of Cardiothoracic Surgery, University of Minnesota, 420 Delaware Street Southeast, MMC 207, Minneapolis, MN 55455, USA
* Corresponding author.
E-mail address: eitanp@umn.edu

Thorac Surg Clin 26 (2016) 333–346
http://dx.doi.org/10.1016/j.thorsurg.2016.04.009
1547-4127/16/$ – see front matter © 2016 Elsevier Inc. All rights reserved.

PATHOPHYSIOLOGY AND CLINICAL PRESENTATION

Normal diaphragm function exerts caudal movement of the diaphragm during inspiration, resulting in expansion of the rib cage, which generates negative intrathoracic pressure and results in lung expansion.[15] In patients with eventration or paralysis, diaphragmatic movement can be diminished, absent, or even paradoxic. As a result, ventilation and perfusion to the basal portion of the lung ipsilateral to the paralyzed or eventrated diaphragm are impaired, the latter possibly caused by regional vasoconstriction induced by alveolar hypoxia[16]; ventilation/perfusion mismatch and loss of chest-wall compliance are among the factors that contribute to dyspnea. Some symptomatic patients develop mild hypoxemia and attempt to compensate by hyperventilating, which can result in mild respiratory alkalosis.[6,17] Others may manifest orthopnea caused by cranial displacement of the affected hemidiaphragm by the abdominal viscera in the supine position, leading to further reductions in lung volumes.[17] A few patients (especially those with left hemidiaphragm eventration) can develop nonspecific gastrointestinal symptoms, such as epigastric pain, bloating, heartburn, regurgitation, belching, nausea, constipation, and weight loss, as the abdominal viscera migrate into the thoracic cavity.[3,7]

DIAGNOSIS AND PREOPERATIVE EVALUATION

Most adults with paralysis or eventration are asymptomatic. Most cases are discovered incidentally on a chest radiograph, showing hemidiaphragm elevation.[4,7]

The diagnosis of symptomatic diaphragmatic eventration or paralysis is mostly clinical, and is based on a focused history and physical examination and a chest radiograph. Dyspnea secondary to eventration or paralysis is predominantly a diagnosis of exclusion. These patients must be evaluated for other primary causes of dyspnea, and if found, corrected or improved if possible (eg, morbid obesity, primary lung disease, heart failure). In patients with dyspnea or orthopnea, a history consistent with hemidiaphragm paralysis (eg, onset of dyspnea after cardiac surgery), and an elevated hemidiaphragm on a standard full-inspiration posteroanterior and lateral chest radiograph, additional diagnostic studies are rarely necessary.

Symptom Evaluation

It is essential to determine the start, duration, and progression of dyspnea and/or orthopnea.

Patients who have diaphragm paralysis can often recall with precision when their dyspnea started or worsened (eg, after cardiac surgery); patients who have eventration may not be able to determine a specific starting point. All patients who have dyspnea secondary to diaphragmatic eventration or paralysis should fill out a standardized respiratory questionnaire to evaluate the severity of their symptoms and to assess their response to treatment.

Objective Respiratory and Quality of Life Evaluation

We use the St George's Respiratory Questionnaire (SGRQ),[18] which is a validated questionnaire that measures health impairment from respiratory disease and quantifies changes in health after therapy. This questionnaire is formed by 2 parts: The first part is a symptoms score that assesses the patient's perception of the frequency and severity of his or her respiratory symptoms. The second part is an activity score, which assesses the degree of impairment of daily physical activities by a respiratory disease, and an effect score, which determines psychosocial dysfunction resulting from respiratory disease. Total scores range from 0 to 100 (normal: 0–6); higher scores translate to worse health impairment. A clinically significant improvement after surgery is defined as a reduction of 4 or more points after an intervention. Other respiratory questionnaires and scales exist, such as the Chronic Respiratory Disease Questionnaire, the Manchester respiratory activities of daily living questionnaire Medical and the Research Council Dyspnea Scale.[19–21] They can be used to objectively measure response to treatments and impact on well-being and quality of life.

Physical Examination

The 2 characteristic findings that may be present on a physical examination in these patients are (1) paradoxic inward movement of the lower costal margin during inspiration (Hoover sign),[22] and (2) abdominal paradox (the rib cage and abdomen move out of phase with each other).[15,23]

Other nonspecific respiratory signs include increased anteroposterior diameter of the chest, diminished maximal excursion of the diaphragm on percussion, and diminished breath sounds on the affected side, mostly at the base.[3,15] If an eventrated diaphragm is exceptionally redundant, a flopping sound may be heard on auscultation.[24]

Pulmonary Function Tests

Standard pulmonary function tests (PFTs) are an unreliable tool to evaluate diaphragm function and do not correlate well with dyspnea in this setting. However, PFTs are essential, as they provide objective evaluation and may identify additional respiratory processes that could be contributing to dyspnea. Diaphragmatic dysfunction decreases chest-wall compliance, and a restrictive pattern is usually seen. Changes observed are a low forced vital capacity (FVC) and low forced expiratory volume in 1 second (FEV1).

As a critical mediator of inspiration, it is important to assess diaphragm function with inspiratory parameters (eg, maximum forced inspiratory flow). FVC should be assessed in the upright and supine position, because supine FVC in healthy individuals can decrease up to 20% from upright values.[25] Furthermore, supine lung volumes may decrease by 20% to 50% when compared with upright values in patients with diaphragmatic eventration or paralysis.[17,26,27] The primary utility of PFTs is to monitor changes over time (eg, after surgery) more than to gage treatment response.

Imaging Studies

Chest radiograph
Preoperative evaluation should include a posteroanterior and lateral (PA/LAT) chest radiograph. On a standard full-inspiration PA/LAT chest radiograph, the right hemidiaphragm is normally 1 to 2 cm higher than the left.[28] In patients with paralysis or eventration, we expect to see an elevated hemidiaphragm. However, this is a nonspecific finding because a variety of pulmonary (ie, atelectasis and fibrosis), pleural (ie, pleural effusions and masses), and subdiaphragmatic processes (ie, hepatomegaly, splenomegaly, gastric dilatation, and subphrenic abscesses) can also cause elevation of a hemidiaphragm.[29] Consequently, further studies may be needed if an elevated hemidiaphragm is noted on a chest radiograph in the presence of dyspnea.

Fluoroscopic sniff test
During fluoroscopy, patients are instructed to sniff and diaphragmatic excursion is assessed. Normally, both hemidiaphragms move caudally. In a positive test, the affected hemidiaphragm paradoxically moves cranially during sniffing. To improve diagnostic specificity, it is required that at least 2 cm of paradoxic motion are noticed during fluoroscopy.[15] A fluoroscopic sniff test is warranted only to confirm the presence of a paralyzed diaphragm when the diagnosis is uncertain. Its ability to distinguish diaphragmatic paralysis (which characteristically demonstrates paradoxic motion during sniffing) from eventration (which usually does not) is of limited value. The decision of whether a patient is a candidate for plication or not should not rely on this test, for various reasons. First, both the paralyzed and the eventrated diaphragm are treated with plication. Second, this test lacks specificity (6% of healthy persons exhibit paradoxic motion on fluoroscopy[30]). Third, patients with eventration may exhibit passive cranial diaphragmatic displacement during the test when sniffing, which can be confused with paradoxic movement. Finally, test interpretation may be difficult. We do not use paradoxic motion as a necessary criterion for diaphragm plication.

Ultrasound
Ultrasound can be used to assess both hemidiaphragms. Parameters evaluated are the thickness and change of thickness of the diaphragm during respiration; studies report up to 80% concordance with fluoroscopy findings.[29,31] Despite this, ultrasound has not been fully validated in clinical practice and its applicability may be hampered by obesity and operator dependency.

Computerized tomography
A computerized tomography scan of the neck, chest, and upper abdomen is useful only to distinguish hemidiaphragm elevation secondary to paralysis or eventration from other causes of phrenic nerve involvement (eg, intrathoracic tumors), subphrenic processes that cause hemidiaphragm elevation, traumatic diaphragmatic hernia, and suspicion of phrenic nerve compression by cervical spinal disease.

Other Diagnostic Tests

Other imaging and functional studies have been used in assessing patients with hemidiaphragm paralysis or eventration. These include dynamic MRI, maximal transdiaphragmatic pressure assessment, and phrenic nerve conduction studies. Dynamic MRI has the advantage of assessing individual segments of the diaphragm during motion in multiple planes. Regardless, these studies have not gained widespread use during the routine clinical evaluation of symptomatic patients with an elevated hemidiaphragm and are of limited practical value.

SURGICAL TREATMENT
Diaphragmatic Plication

Surgical repair of diaphragmatic eventration was first described in 1923.[32] Since then, a variety of open and minimally invasive diaphragm transthoracic and transabdominal plication techniques have been described. Although alternative treatments have been described (eg, diaphragmatic pacing for quadriplegic patients with bilateral diaphragmatic paralysis[33]), they have not gained widespread acceptance.

Indications

The *only* goal of diaphragm plication is to treat dyspnea; hence, operative intervention is indicated *exclusively* for symptomatic patients. An elevated hemidiaphragm or paradoxic motion per se does not warrant surgery in the absence of significant dyspnea.

- Indications for plication are based predominantly on the presence and severity of symptoms (mostly respiratory) and their impact on quality of life
- Dyspnea/orthopnea that cannot be solely attributed to another disease
- An elevated diaphragm that is not caused by another pathologic process other than eventration or paralysis

For adults with phrenic nerve injury (usually thermal) from cardiac surgery, a 1-year to 2-year period of observation is often recommended, as phrenic nerve function may improve with time.[9,10,34,35] However, plication may be warranted after a shorter period of observation (ie, 6 months) if dyspnea is significantly impairing a patient's quality of life or preventing participation in cardiac rehabilitation.

Contraindications

Relative contraindications are as follows:

- Body mass index (BMI) of greater than 35[a]
- Neuromuscular disorders (ie, amyotrophic lateral sclerosis and muscular dystrophy[b])
- Previous upper abdominal operations (for the laparoscopic approach)
- Bilateral hemidiaphragmatic elevation
- A calcified, nonpliable diaphragm

Surgical Approaches

Access to the affected diaphragm can be obtained either through the thorax or the abdomen. Either approach may be done with open or minimally invasive techniques.

Open transthoracic plication

Historically, open transthoracic plication has been the traditional approach to treat symptomatic patients with hemidiaphragm eventration or paralysis. A posterolateral thoracotomy is performed through the sixth,[36,37] seventh,[13,38–40] or eighth[41] intercostal space. A variety of plication techniques have been described, including hand-sewn U-stitches,[36,37,41,42] mattress sutures,[13,39] running sutures with or without pledgets, and stapling[43] techniques with or without mesh.[37,44] Another technique includes resecting the redundant portion of diaphragm and reapproximating the tissue in overlapping layers.[7,45]

Multiple single-institution studies have demonstrated significant improvement in symptoms and respiratory function after open transthoracic plication.[36–38,40,41,46,47] In a study of 17 patients with unilateral paralysis, Graham and colleagues[13] found that an open transthoracic plication led to significant subjective improvement in dyspnea and orthopnea as well as improvement in PFTs (FVC increased by 19% in the upright position and by 42% in the supine position). Five to 10-year follow-up data were available for 6 patients showing sustained improvements in dyspnea scores and PFTs.[13,26] In another study of 19 patients, Higgs[40] demonstrated durable improvements in dyspnea scores and PFTs after open transthoracic plication at 5-year to 10-year follow-up. A more recent report by Calvinho and colleagues[38] in 20 patients operated though a posterolateral thoracotomy demonstrated good results but states that chronic surgical pain can be a

> **Box 1**
> **Operating room preference card**
>
> - General anesthesia
> - Single-lumen endotracheal tube (selective ventilation is not necessary)
> - Supine position
> - Arms abducted
> - Foot board (intraoperative reverse Trendelenburg positioning)
> - Ipsilateral anterolateral chest wall must be included in the operative field for chest tube placement

---

[a]Ideally, morbidly obese patients (BMI >35) should be evaluated for medical or surgical bariatric treatment before plication, because dyspnea may improve after significant weight loss and a plication may no longer be warranted.

[b]Based on our experience and that of others, the benefits of plication on dyspnea in patients with amyotrophic lateral sclerosis or muscular dystrophy are moderate at best, and complications are common.[62] An individualized multidisciplinary approach is necessary to determine if these patients are appropriate candidates for diaphragm plication.

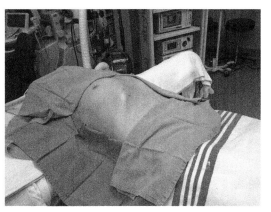

Fig. 1. Patient positioning (supine with arms abducted).

challenge to manage postoperatively. Cumulative experience with open transthoracic plication suggests that plicating the diaphragm for symptomatic eventration or paralysis provides both short-term and long-term benefits. Unfortunately, open transthoracic plication is very invasive, cannot be performed in patients with multiple comorbidities, and chronic pain is often a difficult condition to manage on its own postoperatively. Consequently, alternative approaches to diaphragmatic plication have been developed to minimize the disadvantages of the open transthoracic approach.

Thoracoscopic video-assisted thoracoscopic surgery and robotic-assisted plication

Similarly, a variety of different techniques are described via this approach. Thoracoscopic plication can be performed using 2 ports with a mini-thoracotomy,[48,49] 3 ports,[12,50,51] or 4 ports.[52] Plication techniques include continuous sutures,[49,52] interrupted stitches,[12,51] or stapling.[53] Single-institution studies have reported improvement in dyspnea and PFTs with thoracoscopic plication.[12,48,51] Freeman and colleagues[12] initially reported on 25 patients with hemidiaphragm paralysis in whom thoracoscopic plication was successfully performed in 22 patients, and 3 required conversion to thoracotomy. Follow-up at 6 months demonstrated significant improvement in dyspnea scores and with improvements in FVC (FVC >19%), FEV1 (FFV1 > 23%), functional residual capacity (FRC >21%), and in total lung capacity (TLC >19%). They then reported long-term follow-up (57 ± 10 m) in 41 patients (31 thoracoscopic and 10 thoracotomy) again with demonstrable improvement in PFTs in FVC (17%), FEV1 (21%), FRC (20%), and TLC (20%).[50]

Thoracoscopic robotic-assisted techniques have also been described, one used imbricating rows of horizontal mattress 0-silk sutures.[54–56] Long-term follow-up is not available for plication under robotic technique.

Thoracoscopic diaphragm plication is an excellent minimally invasive alternative to open transthoracic plication; mid-term and long-term follow-up data suggest that it is as effective as the open approach. Workspace limitation by the rib cage and the elevated hemidiaphragm as well as potential for chronic intercostal pain are the main disadvantages of this approach.

Open transabdominal plication

Open transabdominal plication has been described for unilateral or bilateral diaphragmatic eventration or paralysis in the pediatric population.[57] Few outcome data are available on the results of open transabdominal plication in adults. Advantages of an open transabdominal approach are access to both sides of the diaphragm and that it does not require selective ventilation. Additionally, a laparotomy is generally a less morbid incision than a thoracotomy. Disadvantages include an open approach and difficult access to the most posterior portion of the diaphragm.

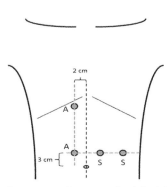
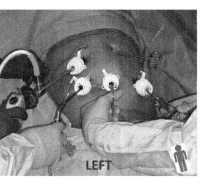
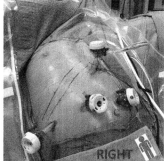

Fig. 2. Port placement for left-sided and right-sided plication.

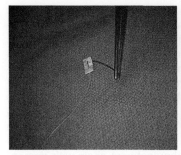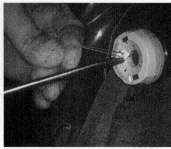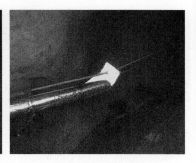

Fig. 3. Technique for intracorporeal use of pledgets.

Laparoscopic plication

Laparoscopic diaphragm plication offers several advantages over the thoracic approaches:

1. Avoids incisions and compression by instruments on the intercostal space, thus avoiding intercostal nerve pain
2. There is no need for selective lung ventilation
3. Excellent visualization can be achieved coupled with ample working space

This technique was initially described by Hüttl and colleagues[58] for 3 patients with symptomatic paralysis of the diaphragm. They reported no intraoperative or postoperative complications or recurrence at a median of 72 months of follow-up, with improvement in symptoms and pulmonary function.

We have previously reported our experience with 25 patients who underwent laparoscopic diaphragm plication.[59] Of the 25 patients, there were 9 right-sided and 16 left-sided plications. Only one conversion to thoracotomy was necessary due to dense intrathoracic adhesion that could not be divided laparoscopically. Five patients had 1 or more complications, including prolonged chest tube drainage (>200 mL/d for 7 days; n = 2),

pleural effusion requiring chest tube placement after discharge from the hospital (n = 1), respiratory failure requiring reintubation (n = 1), upper gastrointestinal hemorrhage (n = 1), stroke (n = 1), urinary tract infection (n = 1), and paroxysmal atrial fibrillation (n = 1). There were no deaths. At 1-year follow-up chest radiograph, the affected diaphragm was lower than before the plication in all patients. We found a significant improvement in the mean SGRQ scores at 1 month following the plication and this improvement was maintained at 1 year. Our patients experienced a more than 20-point reduction in their mean total scores at 1 month and 1-year follow-up. Since that publication, we have performed another 39 laparoscopic diaphragmatic plications for a total of 64 over a 10-year period. Long-term results are being collected for future publication. Based on this, we conclude that laparoscopic diaphragm plication for diaphragm paralysis or eventration is a relatively safe and effective procedure that leads to improved symptoms, respiratory quality-of-life scores, and pulmonary function at mid-term follow-up.

Laparoscopic robotic-assisted techniques have recently been described as a peer-reviewed technical video but without outcome data or short-term results.[60]

Laparoscopic Diaphragm Plication Surgical Technique

Anesthesia

The patient must be under general anesthesia, with a single-lumen endotracheal tube in place (selective ventilation is not necessary).

Position

Supine position, with arms abducted, and with a foot board for intraoperative reverse Trendelenburg positioning. The ipsilateral anterolateral chest wall must be included in the operative field for chest tube placement if necessary (**Box 1**, **Fig. 1**).

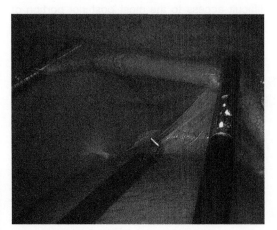

Fig. 4. Takedown of the triangular ligament.

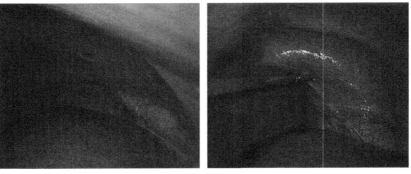

Fig. 5. Small opening on diaphragm (*left*) and floppy diaphragm after equalization of pressures (*right*).

A   **B**

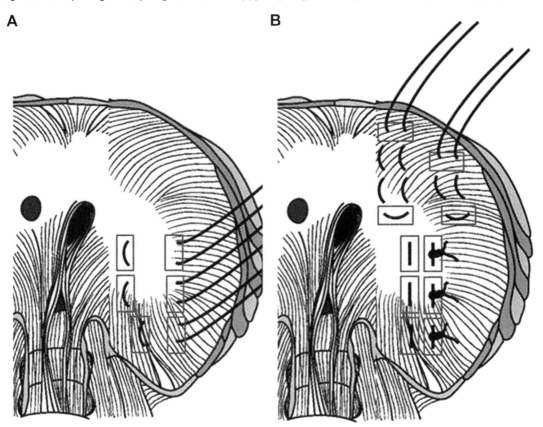

Fig. 6. Schematic of laparoscopic plication stitches. (*A*) Lateral to medial. (*B*) PA.

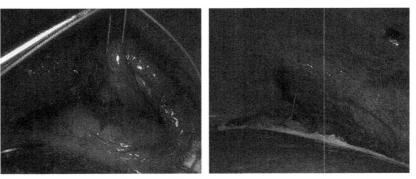

Fig. 7. First posterior stitch as posteriorly as possible mid-distance between the lateral and medial borders of the hemidiaphragms.

Ports

We use four 12-mm ports. Before each port being placed, 0.25% bupivacaine with epinephrine is locally infiltrated for preemptive analgesia. The first port is placed 2 cm above the umbilicus and 2 cm lateral to the midline (contralateral to the diseased diaphragm); the second port is placed near the xiphoid, following a vertical line superiorly from the first port. These 2 ports are used for the 10-mm, 30° camera and the assistant instruments. The third and fourth ports (the surgeon's ports) are placed in a horizontal line 2 cm above the umbilicus, ipsilateral to the diseased diaphragm (**Fig. 2**).

- Four 12-mm ports (see **Fig. 2**)
- Assistant's ports (A): 2 cm parallel to the midline (contralateral to the diseased hemidiaphragm)
- Surgeon's ports (S): placed in a line approximately 2 cm above the level of the umbilicus

Suture material

Our preferred suture material is a #2 braided, nonabsorbable suture (Ti-Cron 36″ double-armed 37-mm needle from Covidien/Medtronic, Minneapolis, MN) with intracorporeal knots. We reinforce all of our stitches with pledgets. Our pledget technique is depicted in **Fig. 3**.

Procedure steps

Exposure We insufflate the abdomen with CO_2 at pressure of 12 to 15 mm Hg and place the patient in steep reverse Trendelenburg position to expose the posterior portion of the hemidiaphragm; transection of the falciform ligament and triangular ligament helps to access the right hemidiaphragm for plication (**Fig. 4**).

Controlled pneumothorax The pneumoperitoneum displaces the thinned-out hemidiaphragm cranially, as a result the hemidiaphragm will be taught and difficult to reach. We make a 5-mm perforation at the dome of the diaphragm with electrocautery (which will ultimately be included in the plication). The resultant pneumothorax allows the hemidiaphragm to flop freely toward the abdominal cavity for grasping and suturing (**Fig. 5**). We alert the anesthesia team for potential hypotension or difficulty ventilating when we perforate the hemidiaphragm, if needed, and we then place a small (<20F) pliable soft chest tube for partial decompression where we slowly vent the pneumothorax intraoperatively, allowing for a low-pressure pneumothorax with minimal cardiopulmonary compromise while keeping the diaphragm floppy.

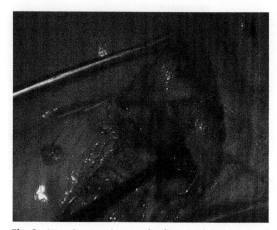

Fig. 8. Anterior traction on the first stitch helps to pull the diaphragm upward and to expose the more posterior aspect for subsequent stitches.

Posterior plication We use interrupted pledgeted U-stitches and first plicate the posterior portion of the hemidiaphragm in an anteroposterior direction. **Fig. 6** represents a schematic of our plication method. We place our first stitch as far posteriorly as possible mid-distance between the lateral and medial borders of the hemidiaphragms (**Fig. 7**). Anterior traction on the first stitch helps to pull the diaphragm upward and to expose the more posterior aspect for subsequent stitches (**Fig. 8**). Usually, we place 3 to 4 stitches anteroposteriorly (**Fig. 9**). This aspect of is technically challenging, as the posterior aspect of the hemidiaphragm is more difficult to access via the abdomen than through the chest. A thorough posterior plication is critical for optimal results.

Anterior plication We place 2 to 3 "weaving" stitches in a posteroanterior direction to plicate the anterior portion of the hemidiaphragm (see

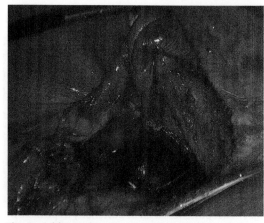

Fig. 9. Additional anteroposterior plicating stitches.

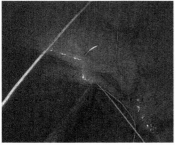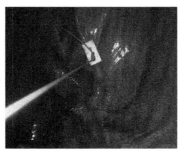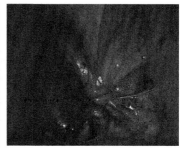

Fig. 10. First weaving PA plicating stitches.

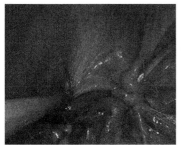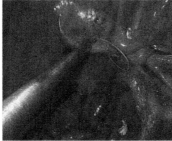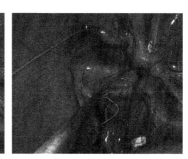

Fig. 11. Second weaving PA plicating stitches.

Table 1 Equipment preference card	
Preference Card	
Equipment	• HD monitor × 2 • Tower video Olympus with Insufflator • Bed attachment extension footboard • Foot pedal for monopolar electrocautery
Instruments	• Laparoscopic cholecystectomy tray • Trocars: 5 mm, 5 mm, 12 mm, 12 mm • Iron intern/Nathanson retractor • Tube scope warming • 5-mm 30 and 45° scope • 10-mm 30° scope • Laparoscopic needle holders • Laparoscopic knot pusher
Positioning devices	• Foot board • Arm boards
Supplies	• 19-Fr Blake drain • Pleurovac • Foley
Sutures	• Pledget PTFE $^1/_2$ × $^1/_4$ × 1/16 inch • Silk #0, SH needle 30 inch × 2 • Silk #2–0, SH needle 30 inch × 1 • Ti-cron #2, GS-21 double-armed needle × 4 • Vicryl 0 Tie 54 inch • Vicryl #4–0 PS-2 needle 18 inch

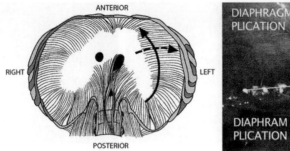
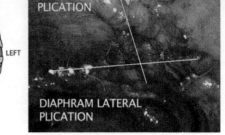

Fig. 12. End results of laparoscopic diaphragmatic plication.

Fig. 6). This portion of the operation is straightforward, as access to the anterior portion of the hemidiaphragm is excellent (**Figs. 10** and **11**). At the end of the operation, the plication should be sufficiently tight, but with care to not add any more plication stitches that could tear the diaphragm. The ultimate result should be a T-shaped plication (**Fig. 12**).

Tube thoracostomy During and at the end of the procedure, we verify that the chest tube has not been trapped with a stitch.

Lung reexpansion At the end of the procedure, we ask the anesthesia team to hand-ventilate several times to peak pressures of 35 to 40 mm Hg to reexpand the atelectatic portion of the lung, followed by ventilation with high tidal volumes and a positive end-expiratory pressure of 10 mm Hg until extubation (**Table 1**).

Postoperative care
Intense pulmonary toilet is mandatory to optimize reexpansion of the ipsilateral lower lobe. We remove the chest tube when the output is less than 200 mL per day. Premature removal can lead to symptomatic pleural effusion. On occasion, patients may be discharged with the chest tube in place if the output is more than 200 mL per day; once the output diminishes, the chest tube can be removed in clinic (approximately 10% of patients will have an elevated chest tube output for more than7 days).

On immediate postoperative chest radiograph, we should observe that the plicated side is lower than the opposite side; one might see elevation of the contralateral hemidiaphragm. At 1 month, both hemidiaphragms are usually seen at approximately the same level (**Fig. 13**).

Complications of diaphragm plication
Reported complications for all approaches include pneumonia, pleural effusions,[59] abdominal compartment syndrome,[61] conversion to open (for minimally invasive approaches),[12,62] abdominal bowel injury,[63] deep venous thrombosis,[50]

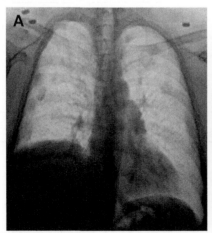
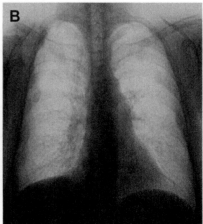

Fig. 13. (*A*) Preoperative PA chest radiograph showing right hemidiaphragmatic elevation. (*B*) PA chest radiograph 1 month after laparoscopic right hemidiaphragm plication; both sides of the diaphragm are at a similar level.

Table 2
Clinical results in the literature

Author	y	n	Laterality	Technique (n)[a] Converted	Questionnaire or Score [Range] (Mean Change)	PFT (% Improvement)	Follow-Up (n)
Graham et al,[13]	1979–1989	17	L = 9, R = 8	Thoracotomy (17)	Dyspnea score [0–10], (−4.1), (−3.4)	FVC (18.5), FVC(17.2)	≥ 6 wk (17), 5 y (6)
Higgs,[40]	1983–1990	19	L = 13, R = 6	Thoracotomy (19)	MRC/ATS grading system [0–4], (−1.3)	FVC (10.1), FEV_1 (11.8), FVC (11.8), FEV_1 (15.4)	Postop (19), Postop, ~10 y, ~10 y
Versteegh et al,[41]	1996–2006	22	L = 10, R = 11, B = 3	Thoracotomy (22)	BDI [0–11] and TDI [−9–+9], (NI)	FVC (13)[a], FEV_1 (10)[a]	~4 y, ~4 y
Mouroux et al,[48]	1992–2003	12	L = 8, R = 4	Thoracoscopy–mini-thoracotomy (12)	NI	FVC (30)[a], FEV_1 (22)[a], FVC (18)[a], FEV_1 (25)[a]	1 y (10), 1 y, 5 y (6), 5 y
Freeman,[12]	2001–2004	25	L = 15, R = 10	Thoracoscopic (25), 3[a]	MRC dyspnea scale [1–5], (−1.9)	FVC (17), FEV_1 (21.4)	6 mo (24), 6 mo
Freeman et al,[50]	2001–2007	41	L = 24, R = 17	Thoracoscopic (30), Thoracotomy (11)	MRC dyspnea scale [1–5], MRADL [max 21],[a] (−2.0), (+7),[a] (−1.9), (+8)[a]	FVC (19), FEV_1 (23), FVC (17), FEV_1 (21)	6 mo, 6 mo, 4 y, 4 y
Hüttl et al,[58]	1994–1998	3	L = 3	Laparoscopic (3)	NI	FEV_1 (8–24)	3 mo (3)
Groth,[59]	2005–2008	25	L = 16, R = 9	Laparoscopic (25), 1[a]	SGRQ (−22.7), (−28.6)	FEV_1 (12.8), FVC (10.3), FIFmax (22.2), FEV_1 (7.4), FVC (3.0), FIFmax (16.2)	1 mo (25), 1 mo, 1 mo, 1 y (25), 1 y, 1 y

Abbreviations: ATS, American Thoracic Society; B, bilateral; BDI, baseline dyspnea index; FEV1, forced expiratory volume in 1 second; FIFmax, maximum forced inspiratory flow; FVC, forced vital capacity; L, left; MRADL, Manchester respiratory activities of daily living; MRC, Medical Research Council; NA, not applicable; NI, no information; Postop, postoperative; R, right; SGRQ, St. George's respiratory questionnaire; TDI, transition dyspnea index.
[a] Values calculated from reported preoperative pulmonary function tests (PFTs) and PFTs at follow-up.

stroke, upper gastrointestinal hemorrhage,[59] pulmonary emboli,[41] arrhythmia,[50] and acute myocardial infarction.[41]

REHABILITATION AND RECOVERY

To assess the response to plication, we reevaluate symptoms with the SGRQ, and repeat PFTs. All patients are systematically evaluated by inpatient physical and respiratory therapists and based on objective assessments we occasionally recommend for additional time in rehabilitation (**Table 2**).

Comparison of Surgical Approaches for Diaphragm Plication

No studies exist comparing the safety and efficacy of different surgical techniques for diaphragm plication. Regardless of technique, the principles of diaphragm plication for symptomatic hemidiaphragm paralysis remain the same and include proper patient selection and a safely performed tight plication. The benefits of minimally invasive over open techniques have been well documented in thoracic and abdominal procedures.[64,65] We advocate that diaphragmatic plication be performed in this fashion, although surgical approach in the end is secondary and a matter of surgeon preference and experience.

SUMMARY

Plication of the diaphragm should be performed on symptomatic patients (with no other explanation for symptoms) with evidence of an elevated diaphragm that is not caused by any other pathologic process besides paralysis or eventration. A variety of open and minimally invasive transthoracic and transabdominal techniques have been described in the international literature. The choice of plication approach is dependent on the expertise of the surgeon. Laparoscopic diaphragm plication for diaphragm paralysis or eventration is a relatively safe and effective procedure that leads to improved symptoms, respiratory quality-of-life scores, and pulmonary function. The surgeon must always exercise meticulous technique, particularly to plicate the posterior portion of the affected hemidiaphragm, when the laparoscopic approach is performed. Improvement in dyspnea is the most important measure of clinical success.

REFERENCES

1. Deslauriers J. Eventration of the diaphragm. Chest Surg Clin N Am 1998;8(2):315–30.

2. Schumpelick V, Steinau G, Schlüper I, et al. Surgical embriology and anatomy of the diaphragm with surgical applications. Surg Clin North Am 2000;80(1): 213–39.

3. Thomas TV. Nonparalytic eventration of the diaphragm. J Thorac Cardiovasc Surg 1968;55(4): 586–93.

4. Chin EF, Lynn RB. Surgery of eventration of the diaphragm. J Thorac Surg 1956;32(1):6–14.

5. Christensen P. Eventration of the diaphragm. Thorax 1959;14:311–9.

6. McNamara JJ, Paulson DL, Urschel HC Jr, et al. Eventration of the diaphragm. Surgery 1968;64(6): 1013–21.

7. Thomas TV. Congenital eventration of the diaphragm. Ann Thorac Surg 1970;10(2):180–92.

8. Riley EA. Idiopathic diaphragmatic paralysis. Am J Med 1962;32(3):404–16.

9. Efthimiou J, Butler J, Woodham C, et al. Diaphragm paralysis following cardiac surgery: role of phrenic nerve cold injury. Ann Thorac Surg 1991;52(4): 1005–8.

10. Curtis JJ, Nawarawong W, Walls JT, et al. Elevated hemidiaphragm after cardiac operations: incidence, prognosis, and relationship to the use of topical ice slush. Ann Thorac Surg 1989;48(6):764–8.

11. Markand ON, Moorthy SS, Mahomed Y, et al. Postoperative phrenic nerve palsy in patients with open-heart surgery. Ann Thorac Surg 1985;39(1): 68–73.

12. Freeman RK, Wozniak TC, Fitzgerald EB. Functional and physiologic results of video-assisted thoracoscopic diaphragm plication in adult patients with unilateral diaphragm paralysis. Ann Thorac Surg 2006;81(5):1853–7.

13. Graham DR, Kaplan D, Evans CC, et al. Diaphragmatic plication for unilateral diaphragmatic paralysis: a 10-year experience. Ann Thorac Surg 1990; 49(2):248–52.

14. Maish MS. The diaphragm. Surg Clin North Am 2010;90(5):955–68.

15. Gibson GJ. Diaphragmatic paresis: pathophysiology, clinical features, and investigation. Thorax 1989;44:960–70.

16. Ridyard JB, Stewart RM. Regional lung function in unilateral diaphragmatic paralysis. Thorax 1976; 31(4):438–42.

17. McCredie M, Lovejoy F Jr, Kaltreider NL. Pulmonary function in diaphragmatic paralysis. Thorax 1962;17: 213–7.

18. Jones PW, Quirk FH, Baveystock CM, et al. A self-complete measure of health status for chronic airflow limitation: the St. George's respiratory questionnaire. Am Rev Respir Dis 1992;145(6):1321–7.

19. Guyatt GH, Berman LB, Townsend M, et al. A measure of quality of life for clinical trials in chronic lung disease. Thorax 1987;42(10):773–8.

20. Bestall JC, Paul EA, Garrod R, et al. Usefulness of the medical research council (MRC) dyspnoea scale as a measure of disability in patients with chronic obstructive pulmonary disease. Thorax 1999;54(7): 581–6.

21. Yohannes AM. Reliability of the Manchester respiratory activities of daily living questionnaire as a postal questionnaire. Age Ageing 2002;31(5):355–8.

22. Hoover CF. The functions of the diaphragm and their diagnostic significance. Arch Intern Med 1913;12: 214–24.

23. Grinman S, Whitelaw WA. Pattern of breathing in a case of generalized respiratory muscle weakness. Chest 1983;84(6):770–2.

24. Michelson E. Eventration of the diaphragm. Surgery 1961;49:410–22.

25. Allen SM, Hunt B, Green M. Fall in vital capacity with posture. Br J Dis Chest 1985;79:267–71.

26. Clague HW, Hall DR. Effect of posture on lung volume: airway closure and gas exchange in hemidiaphragmatic paralysis. Thorax 1979;34(4): 523–6.

27. Gould L, Kaplan S, McElhinney AJ, et al. A method for the production of hemidiaphragmatic paralysis. Its application to the study of lung function in normal man. Am Rev Respir Dis 1967;96(4):812–4.

28. Wynn-Williams N. Hemidiaphragmatic paralysis and paresis of unknown aetiology without any marked rise in level. Thorax 1954;9(4):299–303.

29. Gierada DS, Slone RM, Fleishman MJ. Imaging evaluation of the diaphragm. Chest Surg Clin N Am 1998;8(2):237–80.

30. Alexander C. Diaphragm movements and the diagnosis of diaphragmatic paralysis. Clin Radiol 1966; 17(1):79–83.

31. Houston JG, Fleet M, Cowan MD, et al. Comparison of ultrasound with fluoroscopy in the assessment of suspected hemidiaphragmatic movement abnormality. Clin Radiol 1995;50(2):95–8.

32. Morrison JMW. Eventration of the diaphragm due to unilateral phrenic nerve paralysis. Arch Radiol Electrother 1923;28:72–5.

33. Holder TM. Diaphragm pacing by radiofrequency transmission in the treatment of chronic ventilatory insufficiency: present status. J Thorac Cardiovasc Surg 1973;66:505–20.

34. Summerhill EM. Monitoring recovery from diaphragm paralysis with ultrasound. Chest 2008; 133(3):737–43.

35. Gayan-Ramirez G, Gosselin N, Troosters T, et al. Functional recovery of diaphragm paralysis: a long-term follow-up study. Respir Med 2008;102(5): 690–8.

36. Kuniyoshi Y, Yamashiro S, Miyagi K, et al. Diaphragmatic plication in adult patients with diaphragm paralysis after cardiac surgery. Ann Thorac Cardiovasc Surg 2004;10(3):160–6.

37. Simansky DA. Diaphragm plication following phrenic nerve injury: a comparison of paediatric and adult patients. Thorax 2002;57(7):613–6.

38. Calvinho P, Bastos C, Bernardo JE, et al. Diaphragmatic eventration: long-term follow-up and results of open-chest plicature. Eur J Cardiothorac Surg 2009; 36(5):883–7.

39. Wright CD, Williams JG, Ogilvie CM, et al. Results of diaphragmatic plication for unilateral diaphragmatic paralysis. J Thorac Cardiovasc Surg 1985;90(2):195–8.

40. Higgs S. Long term results of diaphragmatic plication for unilateral diaphragm paralysis. Eur J Cardiothorac Surg 2002;21(2):294–7.

41. Versteegh MIM, Braun J, Voigt PG, et al. Diaphragm plication in adult patients with diaphragm paralysis leads to long-term improvement of pulmonary function and level of dyspnea. Eur J Cardiothorac Surg 2007;32(3):449–56.

42. Schwartz MZ, Filler RM. Plication of the diaphragm for symptomatic phrenic nerve paralysis. J Pediatr Surg 1978;13(3):259–63.

43. Maxson T, Robertson R, Wagner CY. An improved method of diaphragmatic plication. Surg Gynecol Obstet 1993;177(6):620–1.

44. Di Giorgio A, Cardini CL, Sammartino P, et al. Dual-layer sandwich mesh repair in the treatment of major diaphragmatic eventration in an adult. J Thorac Cardiovasc Surg 2006;132(1):187–9.

45. Shah-Mirany J, Schmitz GL, Watson RR. Eventration of the diaphragm. Arch Surg 1968;96:844–50.

46. Ciccolella DE, Daly BDT, Celli BR. Improved diaphragmatic function after surgical plication for unilateral diaphragmatic paralysis. Am Rev Respir Dis 1992;146(3):797–9.

47. Ribet M, Linder J. Plication of the diaphragm for unilateral eventration or paralysis. Eur J Cardiothorac Surg 1992;6(7):357–60.

48. Mouroux J, Venissac N, Leo F, et al. Surgical treatment of diaphragmatic eventration using video-assisted thoracic surgery: a prospective study. Ann Thorac Surg 2005;79(1):308–12.

49. Mouroux J, Padovani B, Poirier NC, et al. Technique for the repair of diaphragmatic eventration. Ann Thorac Surg 1996;62(3):905–7.

50. Freeman RK, Van Woerkom J, Vyverberg A, et al. Long-term follow-up of the functional and physiologic results of diaphragm plication in adults with unilateral diaphragm paralysis. Ann Thorac Surg 2009;88(4):1112–7.

51. Suzumura Y. A case of unilateral diaphragmatic eventration treated by plication with thoracoscopic surgery. Chest 1997;112(2):530–2.

52. Hwang Z. A simple technique for the thoracoscopic plication of the diaphragm. Chest 2003;124(1):376–8.

53. Moon S-W, Wang Y-P, Kim Y-W, et al. Thoracoscopic plication of diaphragmatic eventration using endo-staplers. Ann Thorac Surg 2000;70(1):299–300.

54. Dunning J. Robotic diaphragm plication. Available at: ctsnet.org.

55. Kwak T, Lazzaro R, Pournik H, et al. Robotic thoracoscopic plication for symptomatic diaphragm paralysis. J Robot Surg 2011;6(4):345–8.

56. Ahn J, Suh J, Jeong J. Robot-assisted thoracoscopic surgery with simple laparoscopy for diaphragm eventration. Thorac Cardiovasc Surg 2013; 61(06):499–501.

57. Kizilcan F, Tanyel FC, Hiçsönmez A, et al. The long-term results of diaphragmatic plication. J Pediatr Surg 1993;28(1):42–4.

58. Hüttl TP, Wichmann MW, Reichart B, et al. Laparoscopic diaphragmatic plication: long-term results of a novel surgical technique for postoperative phrenic nerve palsy. Surg Endosc 2004;18(3):547–51.

59. Groth SS, Rueth NM, Kast T, et al. Laparoscopic diaphragmatic plication for diaphragmatic paralysis and eventration: an objective evaluation of short-term and midterm results. J Thorac Cardiovasc Surg 2010;139(6):1452–6.

60. Martin J. Laparoscopic, robot-assisted hemidiaphragm plication. Available at: ctsnet.org.

61. Phadnis J, Pilling JE, Evans TW, et al. Abdominal compartment syndrome: a rare complication of plication of the diaphragm. Ann Thorac Surg 2006; 82(1):334–6.

62. Groth SS, Andrade RS. Diaphragm plication for eventration or paralysis: a review of the literature. Ann Thorac Surg 2010;89(6):S2146–50.

63. Pathak S, Page RD. Splenic injury following diaphragmatic plication: an avoidable life-threatening complication. Interact Cardiovasc Thorac Surg 2009;9(6):1045–6.

64. Paul S, Sedrakyan A, Chiu YL, et al. Outcomes after lobectomy using thoracoscopy vs thoracotomy: a comparative effectiveness analysis utilizing the Nationwide Inpatient Sample database. Eur J Cardiothorac Surg 2013;43(4):813–7.

65. Schlussel AT, Lustik MB, Johnson EK, et al. A population-based comparison of open versus minimally invasive abdominoperineal resection. Am J Surg 2015;209(5):815–23.

Video-Assisted Thoracic Sympathectomy for Hyperhidrosis

Jose Ribas Milanez de Campos, PhD[a],*, Paulo Kauffman, PhD[b],
Oswaldo Gomes Jr, MD[a], Nelson Woloski, PhD[b]

KEYWORDS

- Hyperhidrosis • VATS • Sympathetic denervation • Primary hyperhidrosis
- Thoracic sympathectomy

KEY POINTS

- By the 1980s, open surgery or supraclavicular approach was in use by some groups in sympathetic denervation of the upper limbs with vascular indications.
- Low morbidity, cosmetic results, reduction in the incidence of Horner syndrome, and shortened time in hospital made video-assisted thoracic sympathectomy (VATS) better accepted as a treatment for hyperhidrosis.
- Over the last 25 years, VATS has become routine, leading to a significant increase in the number of papers on the subject in the literature.

INTRODUCTION

The beginning of the 19th century saw improvements in microscopy that allowed Remack[1] to describe histologically the sympathetic ganglia and communicating ramifications; the white and hardened myelinated nervous fibers, and the soft grey matter containing unmyelinated nervous fibers. Toward the end of that century, anatomic and functional investigations allowed for better comprehension of the sympathetic nervous system resulting in the practical application of such knowledge seen in the form of surgical intervention upon the sympathetic system. Initially, sympathectomy was performed empirically to deal with conditions that had no adequate treatment.

The first cervical sympathectomy is attributed to Alexander, who in 1889 treated an epileptic, patient followed by Jonnesco in 1896, who carried out surgical interventions in a large number of epileptic patients. In 1899, Jaboulay resected the lower cervical chain in a patient with exophthalmia and goiter. Failure to achieve success using surgical methods for those conditions as well as for others that had no medical or efficacious surgical alternatives (migraine, kidney pain, and poliomyelitis) led to loss of interest in surgical interventions of the sympathetic nervous system until 1916. It was then that Jonnesco successfully conducted the first clinical application of cervicothoracic sympathectomy on a patient suffering angina bringing pain to a halt. Four years later, Kotzareff adopted the surgical procedure to treat hyperhidrosis for the very first time. By the end of the 1930s, the main indications for cervicothoracic sympathectomy began to take shape, those being hyperhidrosis, thromboangeiitis obliterans, and conditions involving vessel spastics.[2]

The development of thoracoscopy, which was first introduced by Jacobaeus in 1910, allowed Hughes to perform thoracoscopic sympathectomy for the first time in 1942, a method that was later

[a] Department of Thoracic Surgery, University of São Paulo, São Paulo, Brazil; [b] Department of Vascular Surgery, University of São Paulo, São Paulo, Brazil
* Corresponding author. Division of Thoracic Surgery, University of Sao Paulo Medical School, Avenida Albert Einstein 627, 2 Floor, Room 210, Bloco A1, Sao Paulo 05651-901, Brazil.
E-mail address: Jribas@usp.br

Thorac Surg Clin 26 (2016) 347–358
http://dx.doi.org/10.1016/j.thorsurg.2016.04.010
1547-4127/16/$ – see front matter © 2016 Elsevier Inc. All rights reserved.

adopted by Kux to operate on an expressive number of patients publishing his great experience in 1954. Despite the satisfactory results achieved by these authors, and for unknown reasons, the technique did not find international acceptance for more than 30 years.[3]

By the 1980s, endoscopy was in use by some groups in sympathetic denervation of the upper limbs with vascular indications, but it was only in the 1990s that advances in optical systems and instrumentation for thoracic endoscopy made it possible to adopt the technique to perform thoracic sympathectomy as it is known today.[4,5] Low morbidity, good cosmetic results, reduction in the incidence of Horner syndrome, and the shortened time in hospital made video-assisted thoracic sympathectomy (VATS) better accepted by those undergoing treatment for hyperhidrosis. Over the last 25 years, VATS has become routine in the treatment of hyperhidrosis, leading to a significant increase in the number of papers on the subject in the literature.

We considered nowadays that VATS is a definitive and successful treatment option; it is a safe procedure that yields satisfactory results, better quality of life although it still remains associated with compensatory hyperhidrosis (CH), which can occur in virtually all patients with greater or lesser intensity, mainly in the trunk, with unknown physiopathology.[6–8]

PRIMARY OR IDIOPATHIC HYPERHIDROSIS

Primary hyperhidrosis (PH), sometimes referred to as idiopathic hyperhidrosis, is a condition in which there is excessive production of sweat, disproportional to thermoregulation needs. Is typically limited to the palms of the hand, the plantar region, and/or the armpits, and its manifestation is of a symmetric nature. It may also affect the head and face, and often occurs in 2 or more regions of the body. The mechanism underlying PH is not fully comprehended, but it is generally accepted that it results from stimulation of the sympathetic nervous system at its center. What triggers or aggravates PH are either diseases or factors associated with a psychosomatic component. Such conditions can persist well into adulthood, but may also decrease in intensity in some patients as they age. HP affects close to 2.8% of the population and in 12.5% to 56.5% of the patients, there is a positive family history.[9] Weather is not an etiologic factor, but hot damp conditions aggravate perspiration. There are 2 papers reported by Moura Júnior and associates[10] and Garbelin and colleagues,[11] who describe interesting findings in these patients: there is a higher expression of

acetylcholine and alpha-7 neuronal nicotinic receptor subunit in the sympathetic ganglia of patients with PH and the diameter of the thoracic sympathetic chain ganglia is larger than the normal controls. Also, there is a greater number of ganglion cells within the ganglion and a greater number of cells in apoptosis.

Palmar Hyperhidrosis

Palmar hyperhidrosis has been observed to be frequently associated with excessive plantar perspiration and tends to start during childhood, but can become aggravated at adolescence. Its clinical significance is far greater than that wrought by plantar or axillary cases, because palmar hyperhidrosis may lead to marked social, educational, professional, and relationship issues aggravating disturbances of personality that may already be in place. Such individuals wet whatever they touch, hampering writing, reading, and school tasks.[12] From a social and affective point of view, such patients tend to be ostracized, avoiding handshakes, parties, dances, and relationships. Not infrequently do they carry towels about so as to keep their hands dry for at least a while. Palmar symptoms may render a professional incapacitated to perform duties when it comes to handling metals, being called "rusters" owing to the oxidation caused by their sweat. Under such circumstances, those who handle electric or electronic components may even become endangered (**Fig. 1**).

Plantar Hyperhidrosis

Plantar hyperhidrosis often comes associated with palmar symptoms and is thus classified as palmoplantar hyperhidrosis. Less frequently, it has been observed to be associated with axillary hyperhidrosis. The condition is aggravated by footwear made of plastics or rubber that, when tied shut,

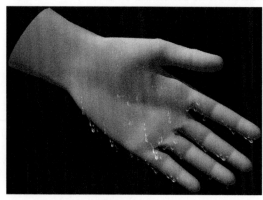

Fig. 1. Palmar hyperhidrosis.

caps evaporation and accentuates perspiration, a scenario certain to lead to skin maceration. Constant humidity promotes conditions for fungal or bacterial infection that cause foul odor not only from the foot itself, but also from socks and shoes.[3] Even wearing open shoes proves to be a challenge because their feet slip within the shoe, losing it at times. Household accidents and those that occur at the workplace or traffic are among other possible outcomes (**Fig. 2**).

Axillary Hyperhidrosis

Axillary hyperhidrosis alone or associated with palmar or plantar or both, most often manifests itself at adolescence, a transitional period known for its great psychological instability associated with hormonal alterations and sexual maturation. Excessive axillary perspiration causes social embarrassment as sweat runs down the body soaking the clothes in its path. An axillary symptom is responsible for individuals refraining from wearing colorful garments, they only use black and white clothes and at times come to the point of embedding an assortment of absorption materials in their armpits throughout daily duties.[13] One noticeable characteristic of such individuals is the fact they are all too often seen wearing either white or black clothes, preferably 1 garment over the other to gingerly disguise the patches of sweat (**Fig. 3**).

Cranial-Facial Hyperhidrosis

Cranial-facial hyperhidrosis is generally observed in adulthood. It too can be a social and

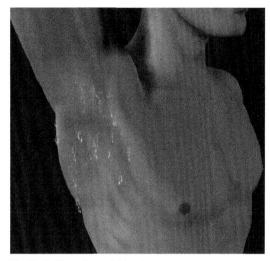

Fig. 3. Axillary hyperhidrosis.

professional embarrassment because it may give the impression of insecurity.[14] It may occur alone or be associated with flushing, a reaction promptly interpreted by others as social phobia. Whether associated or not, both cases may benefit from sympathetic denervation (**Fig. 4**).

THORACIC SYMPATHECTOMY

Until the end of the 1990s and before the use of VATS in medical practice, open chest surgery was the gold standard for cervicothoracic sympathectomy. There are several approaches that can be adopted for that surgery, each with its advantages and disadvantages. For the purpose of

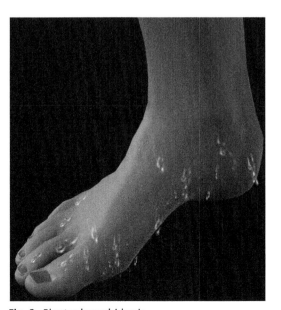

Fig. 2. Plantar hyperhidrosis.

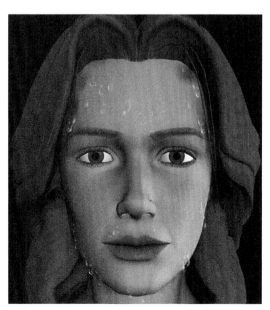

Fig. 4. Craniofacial hyperhidrosis.

cervicothoracic sympathectomy, 3 surgical venues are adopted to reach the area of interest: paravertebral, transthoracic, and supraclavicular. At present, open chest surgery is indicated only when VATS cannot be carried out owing to technical difficulties or in rare cases when there is a concomitant surgical intervention in place like decompression of the thoracic outlet. At present, VATS is considered the gold standard in thoracic sympathectomy, and there are a number of approaches a surgeon may elect to adopt while performing VATS: the 2-, 3-, or 4-door approaches, laterally, dorsally, or an alternative. Each of these are advocated and/practiced according to their advantages and disadvantages. According Campos and Kauffman,[15,16] these authors adopt a practical 2-door technique as described later in this paper.

General Anesthesia

General anesthesia with an endotracheal probe, either simple or of double lumen that enables ventilation to be suspended to achieve the collapse of the lung on the side being operated on. When necessary, bronchoscopy is used to verify the position of the tube. Selective intubation is used mainly in patients who have undergone resection of the fourth ganglia of the thoracic sympathetic chain (G4), or in those individuals with a history of either pleural infection, surgeries, or empyema. Whenever resection is carried out at the second or third ganglia (G2, G3) of the chain a simple light tube can be used in combination with adequate pulmonary ventilation. Long-lasting anesthetics should be avoided to allow for immediate extubation at the end of the procedure.

Positioning

Positioning the patient is placed semiseated on his or her back, the trunk being elevated at 45°. With 2 small cushions under the shoulders to create a space between the armpits and the surgical table, the shoulders are brought forward, thus preventing distention of the brachial plexus that occurs whenever the arms are positioned in abduction at 90°. Another cushion under the knees and a safety belt running over the hips allow the legs to be settled comfortably while preventing their movement on the surgical table when it is tilted laterally, either leftward or rightward, to better expose the surgical sites (**Fig. 5**).

Instruments

Basic equipment includes a thoroscope 5 mm in diameter angled at 30°, a video camera connected to a monitor with a recorder along with a light source, video endoscopic instruments, all measuring 5 mm in diameter, an electrocauterizer (either harmonic or electric), and eventually clips.

Technique

The first incision is made at the height of the fourth or fifth intercostal space, along the anterior axillary line. It is through this slit that the video camera is threaded through into the pleural cavity. The second incision is made at the height of the second and third intercostal space along the medium axillary line and through which the surgical instruments, namely, the electric or harmonic scalpel, scissors, dissection thongs, a retractable hook, and an aspirator, are all placed into proper position within the pleural cavity. In cases where adherence

Fig. 5. Surgical position.

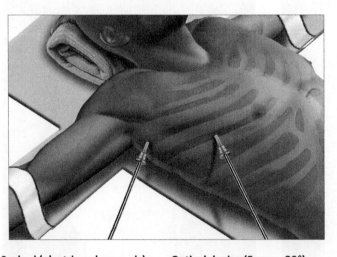

Scalpel (electric or harmonic)   Optical device (5 mm – 30°)
or clip applier

or some technical difficulty is met with, a third incision is made along the posterior axillary line, between the other 2 incisions, to facilitate dissection. A 5-mm trocar is introduced in all incisions that protect the structures of the inner walls of the thorax and keep the passages unimpeded. Insufflation of CO_2 in the pleural cavity was necessary in a few cases to improve surgical access, but most in cases this technique was not adopted or necessary. Once the camera is installed in the pleural cavity, the remaining instruments can then be introduced under plain sight making the procedure safer. The sympathetic chain is identified through the parietal pleura and seen as a whitish, multinodular, longitudinal cordon the forms a slight bulge a little over the heads and costal arches. In elderly patients, or in individuals whose body mass index (BMI) is greater than 26 kg/m^2, the sympathetic chain becomes more difficult to visualize. In such cases, it is identified by means of "palpation" using the surgical instruments. The chain is then identified over the costal arches, always, and the isolated segment is then cauterized. The use of clips on the sympathetic trunk for the purpose of isolating target segments in lieu of thermoablation is an alternative that can be used in some cases, but is certainly not this team's routine practice. Once hemostasis is reviewed a 16-Fr probe attached to an aspirator is placed through the upper trocar and the anesthetist is asked to ventilate the lung until full expansion is achieved.

The video camera and the aspirating probe are subsequently withdrawn and the incision is sutured. Occlusive dressings are left in place over the incisions for 24 hours. In the postanesthetic recovery room, a thoracic radiograph is taken to confirm full lung expansion.

TARGET GANGLIA
Palmar Hyperhidrosis

Early experience with VATS saw physicians resecting extensive segments of the sympathetic chain, including G2 and G3 ganglia (**Fig. 6**), and sometimes reaching the fifth ganglia with satisfactory results. These authors start their experience performing resection at G2 and G3.[3] However, the extent of those resections often resulted in elevated incidence of serious CH and few cases (<1.5%) of Horner syndrome. The team would then perform solely thermoablation, thus limiting intervention only to G2.[14] However, intervention at G2 also resulted in a high rate of CH (64%) owing to the fact denervation occurred over too extensive an area, including cephalic, cervical, and upper limbs segments. Such collateral effects were responsible for 4% of patients regretting having undergone the procedure.[9] Upon conducting a prospective and randomized comparative investigation into the interventions at G2 and G3, these authors realized that the results in both groups were similar and coherent to palmar anidrosis,

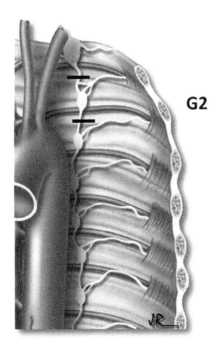
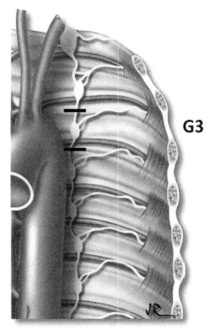

Fig. 6. Examples of G2 and G3.

and that the difference that was observed occurred in the form of intensity of CH, which was significantly less accentuated in patients who had undergone thermoablation at G3.[17] Based on the results of the current study and others in the literature,[12,18,19] we went on to perform thermoablation at G3 when treating palmar hyperhidrosis, and in some special patients with a BMI of greater than 26 kg/m[2], with a tendency to reach G4. That inclination is grounded on results gleaned from our investigations that satisfactory outcomes were verified in the form of reduction of palmar sudoresis, even without achieving anidrosis in many of the patients,[20] as also observed by other authors.[21] The great advantage seen in thermoablation at G4 was the decrease in the intensity of CH when compared with a group of patients treated at G3. In 2001, Lin and Wu[22] stated that the preservation of sympathetic tonus in the cephalic segment offered by intervention limited to G4 would be the main factor responsible for the reduction of such kind of perspiration. Therefore, in patients selected for palmar hyperhidrosis and duly informed, this team has carried out ablation at G4 (these are patients who already have sudoresis in other parts of the body), and who, after having undergone sympathetic denervation at a higher level, may manifest intense CH in those regions, and agree to a possible outcome limited to attenuation of palmar hyperhidrosis, without achieving complete palmar anidrosis.

Axillary Hyperhidrosis

At the beginning of this investigation, we performed resection at G2, G3, and G4. Subsequently, we would spare G2 and perform thermoablation only at G3 and G4 based on what we learned in our ambulatory. More recently, we verified that thermoablation of G4, plain and simple, achieved therapeutic success similar to that seen when there was ablation of G3 and G4 with the advantage of CH being less accentuated, presenting lower recurrence rate, and pushing the patient satisfaction index to greater than 90%.[13]

Cranial-facial Hyperhidrosis and/or Flushing

Sympathetic denervation of the face and head can be achieved by thermoablation of G2, whether it is associated or not with other ganglia. Some authors ventured to resect and/or block from G2 to G4, but few at G5. Following the trend to adhere to only 1 ganglia level, thermoablation at G2 resulted in being the best indication when treating cranial-facial hyperhidrosis with or without flushing.[19,23] In cases of flushing as an exclusive

manifestation, these authors maintain the indication of resection at G2. Despite the greater probability of CH at a level considered high, there does not seem to be an alternative as efficacious for such conditions. Sympathetic blocking at G3 in these patients by means of clips is an alternative recommended by few authors.[24]

Plantar Hyperhidrosis

Although thoracic sympathectomy is not indicated specifically to treat plantar hyperhidrosis that habitually accompanies palmar hyperhidrosis it has proven to be effective in reducing plantar suduresis in 58% of our patients.[7,23,25] The same observation was also related by others.[26-28] The improvements however, are not long lasting, only 24% maintain these results after 1 year.[29] There is not a convincing anatomophysiologic explanation for the improvement; perhaps it is that the greater emotional equilibrium offered by palmar anidrosis achieved by the intervention, at least initially, lessens sympathetic stimuli along the feet venue, with desirable effects on plantar hyperhidrosis. Sympathetic denervation of the feet can be attained by lumbar sympathectomy, which at present, can be performed via retroperitoneal endoscopy. This technique is minimally invasive and has proven to be effective in decreasing plantar sudoresis and improving the quality of life in women with plantar hyperhidrosis who previously underwent VATS for the treatment of palmar hyperhidrosis. Still, 46% of those patients reported worsening of CH in other areas of the body.[30]

ALTERNATIVES TO SYMPATHECTOMY

The ideal treatment for hyperhidrosis is successful, safe, and inexpensive. The growing knowledge of the condition associated with greater patient demand for treatment has allowed for the development of less invasive treatment modalities, with varying effectiveness. Thoracic sympathectomy remains the treatment of choice for patients with hyperhidrosis affecting the palms, axillae, and facial symptoms, presenting improvement in close to 95% of the cases.[31] However, there is a consensus that conservative measures should be tried before progressing to the irreversible effects of surgery. Nonsurgical alternatives for treatment of hyperhidrosis include: topical dermatologic treatments, ionthophoresis, Botox application, and medical therapies.

The main topical dermatologic medication used is aluminum chloride, a topical antiperspirant useful in controlling local hyperhidrosis affecting the palms, soles, and axillae.[32] Drawbacks to this treatment include short-lived effects, skin irritation, and nonadherence, especially in cases of palmar hyperhidrosis, where application can be messy.

Subcutaneous injections of the toxin from the bacterium *Clostridium botulinum* (better known as Botox or Dysport) has been approved by the US Food and Drug Administration for axillary but not for palmar hyperhidrosis. Efficacy is high with this medication, although treatment remains expensive, must be repeated every 3 to 6 months, and is associated with pain ($\sim$50 injections are required in each hand); there may also be anesthesia-related complications.[32]

Oxybutinin is a medical therapy which has been presenting effective results in the control of hyperhidrosis and will be mentioned in the subsequent topic. Sedatives or adrenergic beta-blocker drugs, calcium blockers, and serotonin reuptake inhibitors are medications that may help to reduce social phobia, but do not eliminate hyperhidrosis. These disadvantages are aggravated by the collateral effects they cause. The surgical alternative for treatment of hyperhidrosis include direct axillary sweat gland excision or curettage that are preferred to VATS in some cases because there are fewer systemic effects.

CLINICAL TREATMENT WITH OXIBUTININ

Oxybutynin is an antimuscarinic drug that was first associated with the treatment of hyperhidrosis in 1988. It has recently been reported as an effective initial therapy for adults with excessive sweating, and has been shown to be effective in a randomized, placebo-controlled trial.[33] More recently, short- and long-term results of oxybutynin for hyperhidrosis in children and adolescents have been published, with success in more than 70% to 80% of the patients. With this clinical treatment, we did not observe any worsening of the quality of life; characteristically, when the clinical treatment did not work, quality of life remained unchanged. The use of oxybutynin makes for an attractive therapeutic alternative for the initial treatment of palmar or axillary hyperhidrosis. In choosing this treatment, patients have nothing to lose, and the treatment may facilitate their preparation for facing future invasive procedures. We currently commence treatment of all patients with oxybutynin because it is a worthwhile initial intervention that yields satisfactory results and improves quality of life.[34] In fact, we are also using this clinical treatment to improve screening of the group of patients that will benefit the most with the indication for VATS. We strongly recommend that in all patients.

QUALITY OF LIFE VERSUS PRIMARY HYPERHIDROSIS

Quality of life is presently a meaningful measure in medical practice, and psychosocial factors carry fundamental implications in improving how patients are dealt with. Evaluating quality of life may be performed more easily in cases of serious diseases. In chronic and recurrent cases, and in those whose etiology is complex and saddled with functional, emotional, social, psychological, and professional repercussions, however, such assessments can only be made by means of questionnaires that explore semiobjective criteria that take into account information regarding the patient, the level of discomfort, need to change clothes, as well as the objective verification of the patient.[7]

Thoracic sympathectomy is a therapeutic method capable of markedly altering the quality of life of patients with PH, which can be demonstrated in the questionnaires. Grounded on studies conducted by Amir and colleagues[31] a quality of life questionnaire was developed and applied consecutively in all subjects who had or not been submitted to surgery and/or clinical treatment. The differences between pretreatment and posttreatment assessments were considered "quality of life effects." In short, the questionnaire addresses specific topics, and is easy to be understood and applied, and also assesses alterations in quality of life attributable to sympathectomy in subjects with PH. After the efficacy of the method for the purpose of taming excessive sudoresis, what most counts for such subjects is the occurrence or not of CH, whose intensity may impact results. All patients are and must be thoroughly and exhaustively informed of this possibility.[8,25,28]

This investigation did not make use of any objective gauging of sudoresis because the methods that were available could only produce data at 1 specific point in time. There is no method capable of measuring hyperhidrosis over the entirety of the day. Objective quantification of hyperhidrosis with sudorometers is technically feasible, but these are data that refer to specific times of the day only. Such gauging devices are not portable and data along periods of time throughout the day cannot be collected. The ultimate goal of the questionnaire is the patient's subjective assessment of symptoms. It is the self-reporting method that helps to determine the therapeutic venue indicated for each case. We acknowledge the potential bias when an adult (instead of a child) provides an impression about improvement, but an adult impression of improvement was sought only when the child could not understand and cooperate in the self-assessment. In this setting, we believe self-assessment to be the best, and sometimes the only, option to quantify improvement.[34] After all, PH is disturbing but not dangerous, and the goal of any treatment is the patient's subjective improvement.

RESULTS OF VIDEO-ASSISTED THORACIC SYMPATHECTOMY

Outcomes produced by VATS in the treatment of PH are uniformly good. The immediate aftermath of surgery runs smoothly in most patients who are generally discharged the following day, or at times even on the very same day. The rate of success in achieving anidrosis or reduction of palmar sudoresis is quite high, hovering at 96% to 100% of cases. In axillary hyperhidrosis, that average varies from 83% to 100%, and in crania-facial cases it lies between 87% and 100%. Besides the subjective results, the assessment of quality of life was also considered in the overall evaluation of the subjects scrutinized herein. The objective satisfaction index confronts global results with adverse effects producing "general satisfaction" rates a little under the 85% to 90% range even in children less than 14 years.[35,36]

As mentioned, albeit not specific nor exclusive to the treatment of plantar hyperhidrosis, VATS immediately reduced plantar sudoresis in 50% of the subjects. Still, that benefit did not prove to have long-lasting effects, and after the first year had elapsed from the date of resection, only 24% of the patients continued to enjoy it.[29] Recurrence of palmar or axillary hyperhidrosis has been reported in 1% to 13% in subjects who have undergone resection, and in up to 12% in those with the cranial-facial condition.[2,17] Flushing has proven to be the most challenging clinical condition to be brought under control in our experience. Flushing decreased immediately upon surgical intervention but that improvement does not hold reoccurring with greater or lesser intensity after a few years. Results gleaned from quality of life questionnaires show that 75% to 80% of cases report satisfaction with the treatment, regardless. This team points to some technical failure during the procedure as the reason for such recurrences. A second surgery might be indicated for these cases, notably in precocious ones, and is a venue that meets success. Weak adherence might be verified in such situations, but do not pose as significant hindrances throughout the procedure. Transitory sudoresis of variable intensity may occur along the segment where resection was performed in the first postoperative week, and is observed in 13% of the cases. Such sudoresis

can last for 24 to 36 hours and is caused by the release of neurotransmitters at the terminals of the postganglion sympathetic fibers in degeneration.[23]

Another adverse effect is gustative sudoresis. It differs from those described earlier in that it has been reported in an inconsistent manner, is difficult to characterize, and is seldom reported in the initial postoperative period. Whatever accounts there might be of it are made years after surgery. Gustative sudoresis does not seem to be related to the height of the blockage point along the sympathetic chain. Rather, it is more likely linked to the various diets each region has, and its occurrence ranges from 5.5% to 31.9% of subjects.[25,26] In most cases, it comes in light to moderate intensity and does not interfere with quality of life.

CH is the most often and feared adverse effect of VATS. When intense, it is deemed the greatest cause of patient dissatisfaction.[37,38] CH is characterized by a surge of sudoresis from regions of the body that were previously normal. It occurs mainly on the abdomen, back, and thighs, and becomes uncomfortable when the patient is exposed to heat, stress, agitation, exercise, and closed ambiences. Reports of CH are quite variable as seen in the literature where its occurrence is notified in 35% to 95% of cases depending on what technique was used during the operation. CH may either lose intensity over time or remain the same for years, leaving the patient to learn how to cope with it. There are, however, those who consider CH unbearable, and it is this group that regret having undergone VATS. According to recent studies, whose observations dovetail with what this team has verified over the years, is that there is direct proportion between CH intensity and the extension and height along the sympathetic chain where resection or thermoablation occurs. An explanation for this fact might be found in the damage to afferent fibers responsible for inhibiting perspiration during extensive and higher resections, allowing for more intense manifestations.[39]

Greater BMI also figures as a risk factor for CH. Obese and overweight patients should not be operated on and we consider a BMI of less than 26 kg/m^2 to be suitable for surgery. Despite the fact the literature reports "the higher the BMI the greater compensatory suduresis is," such does not seem to affect the level of satisfaction at first, but after 5 to 10 years, reports appear containing complaints of expressive surges of CH in those whose BMI increased significantly, followed by loss of enthusiasm in answers to inquiries regarding quality of life. In view of these facts, we consider it important to avoid resection or thermoablation at the level of G2 as well as to refrain from resecting extensive portions of the sympathetic chain.[32] A relevant fact that has caught our attention is that the rate of CH was lower, and tolerance to it greater, in children as expressed in their quality of life questionnaires when compared with those of adolescents and adults.[35] Patients must be educated on CH before VATS for PH because of its possible consequences, irreversible nature, and unpredictability.

DIFFICULTIES AND TECHNICAL COMPLICATIONS
Pleural Adherences

Pleural adherences are found quite frequently during endoscopic procedures within the thorax (3%–5%).[2] These are pried loose easily when adherence is weak but firm and extensive adhesions may render VATS unfeasible as in cases of pleural-pulmonary disease when open chest surgery might be the next best option. It is unfortunate that neither routine chest radiographs nor computed tomography scans reveal the existence of adherences before surgery. The clinical history and background of the patient contribute greatly in determining the possibility for adherences and surgical planning, like whenever the anesthetist is asked to perform selective intubation so as to block lung ventilation homolaterally for longer, giving time for the surgeon to pry pleural adherences loose.

The Azygous Lobe

The azygous lobe is an infrequent anatomic variation that hampers VATS. This abnormality, however, in most cases can be detected in chest radiographs before surgery. We have reported 7 successful surgical cases, but in practically all procedures the identification of the chain and access to the upper ganglia was attained once the pleural sheathing that grows around the azygous vein was cut through, allowing that vein to be pushed aside allowing access to the chain from below and medially.[16]

Significant Hemorrhage

Significant hemorrhage during surgery is rare, and when it does occur it is attributed to vessel ruptures or lesions to intercostal vessels during resection chain. Bleeding can also occur at the incision points where the trocar is placed as reports of laceration of the subclavii artery and pseudoaneurysm of the intercostal artery were reported in the literature in a case that required emergency thoracotomy. Such events are fortunately rare in the hands of seasoned professionals, particularly with the techniques in place for thoracic surgery.

Chylothorax

Chylothorax is a very rare condition that results from laceration of the vessels and/or of the thoracic canal. In almost all cases, it has been described in the literature its occurrence was on the left side and in surgical procedures that required extensive manipulation and/or dissection in the proximity of sympathetic ganglia G4 and G5. Despite the extensive and varied distribution of lymphatic vessels all along the thoracic duct, it is at these heights close to where the thoracic duct transverses from the right hemithorax to the left one to begin its ascent until it meets the subclavian vein. Dissections at this anatomic point must be more delicate and minimal, painstakingly identifying and resecting sympathetic tissue strictly limited to this site.

Pneumothorax

Pneumothorax is the most common complication during surgery. Most patients (75%) carry a small amount of residual air or gas left after surgery, and drainage is only needed in a small percentage of those cases 0.4% to 2.3%.[9] Very rarely does hypertensive pneumothorax occur during VATS, but it may happen as a consequence of either a direct lesion to the lung inflicted when inserting the trocars, a lesion to the parenchyma in atypical adherence when there is a collapsed lung, or even more rarely, in iatrogenic lesions. Atypical blisters may occasionally be found and these may burst under the higher pressures at the time of lung insufflation. Surgical measures can be taken ad hoc to correct such events and we strongly recommend postoperative radiographs to confirm the possibility of pneumothorax and the full expansion of the lung.[40]

Subcutaneous Emphysema

Subcutaneous emphysema confined to the thoracic wall and in the vicinity of the point of trocar insertion is a rare occurrence in 2% of patients. Conservative treatment is adopted in most cases when it is unassociated with pneumothorax.[9]

Pulmonary Atelectasis

Pulmonary atelectasis may also occur occasionally, especially in the upper lobes (under 1.2% of patients). Postoperative treatment is respiratory physiotherapy, but this can well be done without, provided the anesthetist efficiently expands the lung at the end of the procedure.[2]

Transitory Brachycardia

Transitory brachycardia during VATS also figures as a rare occurrence during the surgical procedure, and full recovery is observed in practically all patients after a few minutes under clinical observation. Whenever recovery is not so promptly achieved, brachycardia ceases within 2 weeks' time.[2] Heart arrest during VATS for hyperhidrosis has been reported only twice in the literature, and in both cases reanimation was successful. Precaution and a full cardiac evaluation should be performed, particularly in those who have a history of brachycardia and/or prior arrhythmia.[41]

Postoperative Pain

Postoperative pain is a frequent complaint, and is manifested acutely for some hours when taking deep breaths, particularly at the end of inhalation. This symptomology can be treated with analgesics and antiinflammatories that should be administered throughout the first postoperative week for the comfort of those patients. However, there are different approaches; some investigators reported that a thoracoscopic, internal intercostal nerve block with bupivacain 0.5% during VATS is safe and effectively reduced immediate postoperative pain as well as analgesic requirements.[42]

Paresis and Paresthesia

Paresis and paresthesia of the upper limbs were observed in some patients in our early work with VATS owing to the position of the arms on the surgical table, elevated and immobilized in an arch, which may have been the cause of distention of the brachial plexus. In all patients, the manifestations described herein recoiled within a period ranging from 3 days to 3 weeks. After adopting the position described herein, we no longer experienced with this kind of complication.[43]

Horner Syndrome

Horner syndrome is a condition that occurs when there is complete sympathetic denervation of an upper limb, reaching the stellate ganglion. Our practice only observed this complication in 4 cases when members of this team acted on the second thoracic ganglia using an electric scalpel to cauterize the sympathetic chain. In 2 of those cases, the syndrome was transitory, with total resolution toward the end of the second month, and in the remaining 2 cases resolution was permanent. The syndrome is caused by direct or indirect lesion to the stellate ganglion. Temperature from above caused by the electric scalpel when performing ablation of G2 is responsible for the onset of the syndrome. The condition has no longer been observed because we rarely act on the second ganglia at present, and even in the few cases we do the ultrasonic scalpel rather than the hotter electric one is used, which has now become the instrument of choice to perform thermoablation of the sympathetic chain. Horner syndrome may also occur when the sympathetic chain suffers excessive traction during thermoablation.[3]

Contraindications

Contraindications to VATS, could be considered when there is pulmonary infection in course with plural leakage that requires either puncturing or draining, previous pulmonary disease like tuberculosis that cause dense pleural adherence, previous extensive thoracic surgery like pneumonectomy or lobectomy, thoracic radiotherapy, sinus brachycardia, hematologic conditions, and different clinical conditions like Takayasus arteritis, with a lot of alterations in the upper limbs arterial branches and also in which endotracheal anesthesia is contraindicated. High BMI and obesity are also factors deemed that we considered relevant in the contraindication of VATS although same of overweight patients report an increased rate of satisfaction with the surgery.

REASONS FOR VIDEO-ASSISTED THORACIC SYMPATHECTOMY FAILURE
Incomplete Surgery

There are few scenarios that may lead to the inefficacy of VATS, and incomplete denervation figures as one of the main reasons. It occurs when the surgeon fails to correctly identify the target structures and does not perform full thermoablation on them. Inadequate blockage of the sympathetic chain by means of clips also leads to failure. Even when the surgical procedure is correct, failure may occur late into the surgery owing to activation of intermediary ganglia (microscopic clusters of ganglion cells distributed along the communicating pathways or even in the anterior roots of cervical and brachial nerves). We reoperated on 16 patients in our early experience from a total of 2000 cases treated surgically owing to recurrent symptoms. These were found to have been caused by incomplete denervation and were the main reason for the failure of VATS in those cases. Fifteen of these patients underwent complementary thermoablation at the correct levels, which resulted in therapeutic success.[44]

Regeneration

To date, there is no evidence of proven regeneration of sympathetic ganglion cells once the ganglia is removed as their axons degenerate. However, if only the axis-cylinder is severed new fibers may regenerate sprouting from the ganglion cell.[45] Such event may impact surgeries in which paravertebral ganglia are not fully resected and/or blocked.

Functional Reorganization

The sprouting theory was first raised by Murray and Thompson in 1957 as an attempt to explain the resumption of neural activity subsequent to preganglia sympathectomy in the upper extremities. The theory postulates that degenerating fibers produce humoral substances that would stimulate intact nerve fibers to establish connections with nearby sympathetic ganglia.[46] Thus, sectioning the preganglia fibers responsible for innervation of the upper limbs would give the fibers that travel through the stellate ganglion on their way to the upper cervical ganglion favorable conditions to establish connections to that ganglion by sprouting. Besides, there could be connections between these ramifications and the ganglia cells present in spinal nerves, which would explain resumption of sympathetic activity in that limb.

REFERENCES

1. Andres KH, von Düring M, Jänig W, et al. Degeneration patterns of postganglionic fibers following sympathectomy. Anat Embryol (Berl) 1985;172(2):133–43.
2. Wolosker N, Kauffman P. Thoracic sympathectomy. In: Rutherford R, editor. Vascular surgery. 7th edition. Philadelphia: Saunders; 2010. p. 1854–64.
3. Kauffman P, Milanez JRC, Jatene F, et al. Simpatectomia cervicotorácica por vídeotoracoscopia: Experiência inicial. Rev Colégio Brasileiro de Cirurgiões 1998;25:235–9.
4. Strutton DR, Kowalski JW, Glaser DA, et al. US prevalence of hyperhidrosis and impact on individuals with axillary hyperhidrosis: results from a national survey. J Am Acad Dermatol 2004;51:241.
5. Krasna MJ. Thoracoscopic sympathectomy: a standardized approach to therapy for hyperhidrosis. Ann Thorac Surg 2008;85:S764.
6. Wolosker N, Yazbek G, Ishy A, et al. Is sympathectomy at T4 level better than at T3 level for treating palmar hyperhidrosis? J Laparoendosc Adv Surg Tech A 2008;18:102.
7. De Campos JR, Kauffman P, Wolosker N, et al. Quality of life, before and after thoracic sympathectomy: report on 378 operated patients. Ann Thorac Surg 2003;76:886.
8. Teivelis MP, Varella AY, Wolosker N. Expanded level of sympathectomy and incidence or severity of compensatory hyperhidrosis. J Thorac Cardiovasc Surg 2014;148(5):2443–4.
9. Cerfolio RJ, De Campos JR, Bryant AS, et al. The Society of Thoracic Surgeons expert consensus for the surgical treatment of hyperhidrosis. Ann Thorac Surg 2011;91(5):1642–8.
10. Moura Júnior NB, das-Neves-Pereira JC, de Oliveira FR, et al. Expression of acetylcholine and its receptor in human sympathetic ganglia in primary hyperhidrosis. Ann Thorac Surg 2013;95(2):465–70.
11. Oliveira FR, Moura NB Jr, de Campos JR, et al. Morphometric analysis of thoracic ganglion neurons in subjects with and without primary palmar hyperhidrosis. Ann Vasc Surg 2014;28(4):1023–9.
12. Yoon DH, Ha Y, Park YG, et al. Thoracoscopic limited T-3 sympathicotomy for primary hyperhidrosis: prevention for compensatory hyperhidrosis. J Neurosurg 2003;99(Suppl 1):39–43.
13. Munia MA, Wolosker N, Kauffman P, et al. A randomized trial of T3-T4 versus T4 sympathectomy for isolated axillary hyperhidrosis. J Vasc Surg 2007;45:130.
14. Lin TS, Wang NP, Huang LC. Pitfalls and complication avoidance associated with transthoracic endoscopic sympathectomy for primary hyperhidrosis (analysis of 2200 cases). Int J Surg Investig 2001;2:377.
15. Campos JRM, Kauffman P. Simpatectomia torácica por videotoracoscopia para tratamento da hiperidrose primária. J Bras Pneumol 2007;33(3):xv–xvii/editorial.
16. Kauffman P, Wolosker N, de Campos JR, et al. Azygos lobe: a difficulty in vídeo-assisted thoracic sympathectomy. Ann Thorac Surg 2010;89:e57–9.
17. Yazbek G, Wolosker N, de Campos JR, et al. Palmar hyperhidrosis – which is the best level of denervation using video-assisted thoracoscopic sympathectomy: T2 or T3 ganglion? J Vasc Surg 2005;42(2):281–5.
18. Yoon SH, Rim DC. The selective T3 sympathicotomy in patients with essential hyperhidrosis. Acta Neurochir (Wien) 2003;145(6):467–71.
19. Dewey TM, Herbert MA, Hill SL, et al. One year follow-up after thoracoscopic sympathectomy for hyperhidrosis: outcomes and consequences. Ann Thorac Surg 2006;81:1227–32.
20. Wolosker N, Varella AY, Teivelis MP, et al. Regarding optimal level of sympathectomy for primary palmar hyperhidrosis: T3 versus T4 in a retrospective cohort study. Int J Surg 2014;12(8):788.
21. Neumayer C, Panhofer P, Zacherl J, et al. Effect of endoscopic thoracic sympathetic block on plantar hyperhidrosis. Arch Surg 2005;140:676–80.
22. Lin CC, Wu HH. Endoscopic t4-sympathetic block by clamping(ESB4) in the treatment of hyperhidrosis palmaris et axillaris – experience of 165 cases. Ann Chir Gynaecol 2001;90:167–9.

23. Kauffman P, de Campos JRM, Wolosker N, et al. Thoracoscopic cervicothoracic sympathectomy: an eight-year experience. Braz Vasc Surg 2003;2:22–8.

24. Neumayer C, Zacherl J, Holak G, et al. Experience with limited endoscopic thoracic sympathetic block for hyperhidrosis and facial blushing. Clin Auton Res 2003;13(Suppl 1):152–7.

25. Campos JRM, Kauffman P, Kang DWW. Simpatectomia torácica no tratamento da hiper-hidrose primária. In: Moraes IN, editor. Tratado de Clínica Cirúrgica. São Paulo (Brazil): Roca; 2005. p. 1015–9.

26. Chen HJ, Shih DY, Fung ST. Transthoracic endoscopic sympathectomy in the treatment of palmar hyperhidrosis. Arch Surg 1994;129:630–3.

27. Hederman WP. Present and future trends in thoracoscopic sympathectomy. Eur J Surg Suppl 1994;572: 17–9.

28. Doolabh N, Horswell S, Williams M, et al. Thoracoscopic sympathectomy for hyperhidrosis: indications and results. Ann Thorac Surg 2004;77:410–4.

29. Wolosker N, Yazbek G, Milanez de Campos JR, et al. Evaluation of plantar hyperhidrosis in patients undergoing video-assisted thoracoscopic sympathectomy. Clin Auton Res 2007;17(3):172–6.

30. Loureiro Mde P, de Campos JR, Kauffman P, et al. Endoscopic lumbar sympathectomy for women: effect on compensatory sweat. Clinics (Sao Paulo) 2008;63(2):189–96.

31. Campos JRM, Kauffman P, Werebe EC, et al. Questionário de qualidade de vida em pacientes com hiperidrose primária. J Pneumol 2003;29(4):178–81.

32. Campos JRM, Wolosker N, Takeda FR, et al. The body mass index and level of resection. Predictive factors for compensatory sweating after sympathectomy. Clin Auton Res 2005;15:116–20.

33. Wolosker N, de Campos JR, Kauffman P, et al. A randomized placebo-controlled trial of oxybutynin for the initial treatment of palmar and axillary hyperhidrosis. J Vasc Surg 2012;55(6):1696–700.

34. Wolosker N, Teivelis MP, Krutman M, et al. Long-term results of oxybutynin treatment for palmar hyperhidrosis. Clin Auton Res 2014;24(6):297–303.

35. Neves S, Uchoa PC, Wolosker N, et al. Long-term comparison of video-assisted thoracic sympathectomy and clinical observation for the treatment of palmar hyperhidrosis in children younger than 14. Pediatr Dermatol 2012;29(5):575–9.

36. Kao MC, Chen YL, Lin JY, et al. Endoscopic sympathectomy treatment for craniofacial hyperhidrosis. Arch Surg 1996;131(10):1091–4.

37. Kim do H, Hong YJ, Hwang JJ, et al. Topographical considerations under video-scope guidance in the T3,4 levels sympathetic surgery. Eur J Cardiothorac Surg 2008;33(5):786–9.

38. Libson S, Kirshtein B, Mizrahi S, et al. Evaluation of compensatory sweating after bilateral thoracoscopic sympathectomy for palmar hyperhidrosis. Surg Laparosc Endosc Percutan Tech 2007;17:511.

39. Lyra RM, Campos JRM, Kang DW, et al. Sociedade Brasileira de Cirurgia Torácica. Guidelines for the prevention, diagnosis and treatment of compensatory hyperhidrosis. J Bras Pneumol 2008;34(11): 967–77.

40. Lima AG, Marcondes GA, Teixeira AB, et al. The incidence of residual pneumothorax after video-assisted sympathectomy with and without pleural drainage and its effect on postoperative pain. J Bras Pneumol 2008;34(3):136–42.

41. Lin CC, Mo LR, Hwang MH. Intraoperative cardiac arrest: a rare complication of T2,3-sympathicotomy for treatment of hyperhidrosis palmaris. Two case reports. Eur J Surg Suppl 1994;(572):43–5.

42. Bolotin G, Lazarovici H, Uretzky G, et al. The efficacy of intraoperative internal intercostal nerve block during video-assisted thoracic surgery on postoperative pain. Ann Thorac Surg 2000;70(6): 1872–5.

43. Campos JRM, Kauffman P, Wolosker N, et al. Axillary hyperhidrosis: T3/T4 versus T4 thoracic sympathectomy in a series of 276 cases. J Laparoendosc Adv Surg Tech A 2006;16:598–603.

44. Ramsaroop L, Singh B, Moodley J, et al. Anatomical basis for a successful upper limb sympathectomy in the thoracoscopic era. Clin Anat 2004;17(4):294–9.

45. Goetz RH. Sympathectomy for the upper extremities. Chapter 25. In: Dale WA, editor. Management of arterial occlusive disease. Chicago: Year book medical publishers; 1971. p. 431–45.

46. Murray JG, Thompson JW. Collateral sprouting in autonomic nervous system. Br Med Bull 1957;13:213.

Current Treatment of Mesothelioma

Extrapleural Pneumonectomy Versus Pleurectomy/Decortication

Andrea S. Wolf, MD, MPH, Raja M. Flores, MD*

KEYWORDS

- Malignant pleural mesothelioma • Extrapleural pneumonectomy • Pleurectomy decortication

KEY POINTS

- Extrapleural pneumonectomy (EPP) entails en bloc resection of the lung, parietal and visceral pleurae, diaphragm, and pericardium.
- Pleurectomy decortication (P/D), either radical or extended, removes the parietal and visceral pleurae, including resection of the diaphragm and/or pericardium if involved, but preserves the underlying lung.
- Thorough preoperative evaluation of the patient's physiology allows for appropriate intraoperative decisions regarding EPP versus P/D.
- P/D is associated with better short-term outcomes than EPP in the form of perioperative morbidity and mortality.

INTRODUCTION

Although controversial, the role of surgical resection in malignant pleural mesothelioma (MPM) is based on the principle of macroscopic resection of a solid tumor with adjuvant therapy to treat micrometastatic disease. Cancer-directed surgery for MPM is associated with a 5-year survival rate of 15%.[1–3] Two operations have been developed in this context: (1) extrapleural pneumonectomy (EPP), which involves the en bloc resection of the lung, parietal and visceral pleurae, diaphragm, and pericardium; and (2) radical or extended pleurectomy/decortication (P/D), which involves removal of the parietal and visceral pleurae, including resection of the diaphragm and/or pericardium if involved with tumor, but always preservation of the underlying lung. Various patient-specific and even surgeon-specific or center-specific factors may influence which operation is performed. Most studies evaluating the surgical treatment of MPM have focused exclusively on either EPP or P/D, performed as part of multimodality therapy with numerous adjuvant treatments, including preoperative or postoperative chemotherapy, intracavitary chemotherapy or photodynamic therapy, preoperative or postoperative external beam radiation, and now immunologic therapy.[4–9] Results of single-center studies have been biased in favor of one or the other procedure and, consequently, there has been little evidence driving the decision of which operation to perform for individual patients.

Conflict of Interest: The authors have nothing to disclose.
Department of Thoracic Surgery, Mount Sinai Health System, Icahn School of Medicine at Mount Sinai, One Gustave L. Levy Place, Box 1023, New York, NY 10029, USA
* Corresponding author.
E-mail address: raja.flores@mountsinai.org

thoracic.theclinics.com

THE CASE FOR SURGERY IN TREATMENT OF MALIGNANT PLEURAL MESOTHELIOMA

Although there is no defined standard treatment for MPM, most studies in the literature support the use of curative intent surgery in the context of multimodality therapy.[10–13] Surgical resection is offered to more than 40% of MPM patients seen at large tertiary referral centers.[14] In the general population, however, fewer patients are offered cancer-directed surgery. Flores and colleagues[15] reported that cancer-directed surgery was performed in only 22% of 5937 patients with MPM in the Surveillance, Epidemiology and End Results (SEER) dataset between 1990 and 2004. Patients who underwent surgery experienced a median overall survival of 11 months (compared with 7 months without, $P<.0001$) and cancer-directed surgery was an independent predictor of improved survival (hazard ratio, 0.68; 95% CI, 0.63–0.74). In a more recent comprehensive SEER analysis of 13,734 white and black MPM patients diagnosed between 1973 and 2009, cancer-directed surgery was predictive of longer survival.[1]

Left untreated, the median overall survival of patients with MPM is 7 months.[11] Many clinicians support treatment with surgery-based multimodality therapy for patients with favorable disease characteristics. Prognostic factors associated with longer survival are epithelial histology, female gender, and earlier stage. In 1 retrospective study of 945 patients, epithelial histology, female gender, earlier stage, lack of smoking or asbestos exposure, and left-sided disease were associated with longer survival.[16] Women experience longer survival compared with men, but this finding has been more consistent for younger women and those with epithelial tumors. Women under the age of 50 with early stage MPM demonstrated a median survival of greater than 30 months in a retrospective study of patients undergoing EPP for MPM.[10] In another SEER analysis of 14,229 MPM patients diagnosed in the United States between 1973 and 2009, female gender was a significant predictor of longer survival, independent of age, stage, race, and treatment (adjusted hazard ratio, 0.78; 95% CI, 0.75–0.82).[12] For men and women, higher stage disease and nonepithelial histology are associated with lesser survival.[10,16]

OPTIONS FOR SURGERY
Extrapleural Pneumonectomy

Irving Sarot[17] first described the surgical technique of EPP in his mid-20th century case series of patients with tuberculosis treated at the Mount Sinai Hospital in New York City. Butchart and colleagues[18] published the first series of EPP as treatment for patients with MPM in 1976, with a perioperative mortality rate of 31%. Butchart and associates emphasized that this technique may be indicated for certain types of tumors and, thus, adequate preoperative cardiopulmonary evaluation and careful perioperative management of patients were mandated.

In the decades that followed Butchart and coworkers' series, improvements in patient preoperative risk stratification, operative technique, anesthesia, monitoring, and early identification of complications reduced the mortality of EPP to rates less than 4%.[2,19] Modern series describing results of EPP for MPM report postoperative mortality of 2.2% to 7%.[11,20–23]

Preoperative evaluation for extrapleural pneumonectomy

Patients diagnosed with MPM who are considered for EPP are staged with PET computed tomography to evaluate for nodal or distant metastases. The level of PET avidity of the pleural tumor has been shown to correlate with survival, with greater avidity associated with lesser survival.[24] Enlarged and/or PET-avid mediastinal lymph nodes are evaluated with endobronchial ultrasonography or cervical mediastinoscopy. Although some centers perform routine staging mediastinoscopy in all patients, others have abandoned this because of the variable nodal drainage of the pleura with unpredictable pattern of nodal metastases and the lack of sensitivity of cervical mediastinoscopy for detecting extrapleural nodal spread in MPM.[25,26] Chest MRI is often performed to evaluate for diffuse chest wall, transdiaphragmatic, or transmediastinal invasion of tumor.[27] The presence of transdiaphragmatic extension of tumor and/or ascites warrants further evaluation with staging laparoscopy because intraabdominal tumor would preclude surgical resection.

The remaining preoperative evaluation is to determine the patient's ability to tolerate EPP.[11] Pulmonary function tests, including spirometry and diffusion lung capacity, should be performed. Quantitative ventilation/perfusion scan ("split function" test) is routinely done to assess perfusion to the affected lung. The product of the proportion of perfusion to the contralateral lung (which will remain after pneumonectomy) and the forced expiratory volume in 1 second is the predicted postoperative forced expiratory volume in 1 second. Although many clinicians recommend a value of at least 800 mL for pneumonectomy, the added morbidity of extrapleural, diaphragmatic, and pericardial resection have led most surgeons to consider a higher level, such as 1.2 L, for all but the smallest patients.[21] Both a stress test to rule out inducible myocardial ischemia from coronary artery disease and an echocardiogram with Doppler estimation of pulmonary artery pressure based on tricuspid regurgitation should also be performed. A patient with preexisting pulmonary hypertension may not survive the added right ventricular strain of pneumonectomy. Finally, duplex ultrasound of the lower extremity veins to rule out deep vein thrombosis, particularly in patients who have undergone neoadjuvant therapy, is performed. MPM patients have a high incidence of occult deep vein thrombosis and preoperative treatment with anticoagulation (and possibly inferior vena cava filter) may reduce the risk of fatal pulmonary embolus after pneumonectomy.

Extrapleural pneumonectomy perioperative management

Preparation for EPP by the anesthesiologist includes placement of routine monitors, lines, and an epidural catheter for perioperative regional pain control.[28] An arterial line is needed owing to rapid hemodynamic changes and large-bore intravenous access, including a central line, is recommended. If there is any concern regarding pulmonary hypertension, a Swan-Ganz catheter is floated with caution to pull this back before pulmonary artery division. Central lines should be placed on the operative side to avoid pneumothorax on the side of the ventilated (and postoperatively, only) lung. Lung isolation may be obtained with double-lumen endotracheal tube (preferred) or bronchial blocker, with the latter to be pulled back before division of the bronchus. Finally, a nasogastric tube is inserted to aid in identifying the esophagus intraoperatively and to decompress the stomach postoperatively. The disruption of vagal fibers to the bronchus often causes mild postoperative esophageal dysmotility and nasogastric decompression may prevent life-threatening aspiration after pneumonectomy in the early postoperative period.

Extrapleural pneumonectomy surgical technique

Although the detailed steps may vary by surgeon, the basic technique of EPP is consistent. An extended posterolateral thoracotomy, incorporating prior incisions if possible, is performed, usually resecting the sixth rib. The tumor is separated from the endothoracic fascia by dissecting in the extrapleural plane. Dissection is continued posteriorly, anteriorly, superiorly, and inferiorly. The posterior borders of dissection are the azygous vein on the right and the aorta on the left. Caution not to dissect beyond these borders is necessary to avoid avulsion of the azygous vein/tributaries or intercostal aortic branches.

Apically, the subclavian vessels must be identified to avoid injury. As the dissection is continued down the superior mediastinum, the superior vena cava on the right and the aortic arch on the left are at risk. Anteriorly, the thymic fat and pericardium are the border for dissection. The anterior pericardium is incised and the inner surface is palpated for evidence of tumor invasion. A large pericardial effusion unexpectedly encountered at this point warrants even more cautious inspection because it is suggestive of transpericardial invasion.

If no invasion of critical mediastinal structures is identified, the dissection continues. The anterior pericardial incision is continued inferiorly to the medial border of the diaphragm. The diaphragmatic attachments to the chest wall are dissected bluntly with the fingers or with the aid of the Cobb. On the right, caution is exercised in the area of the inferior vena cava deep in the costophrenic recess posteriorly as the inferior pulmonary ligament is divided. On the left, a rim of diaphragmatic crus is retained to decrease the risk of postoperative gastric herniation. Phrenic vessels are clipped and/or coagulated as the diaphragm is resected. The pericardial incision is continued posteriorly and continued superiorly to divide the remaining posterior pericardium.

The hilum is approached last to complete the resection. The superior and inferior pulmonary veins are divided within the pericardium. The right pulmonary artery is divided within the pericardium but, on the left, the intrapericardial segment of pulmonary artery is very short, and the artery is generally divided extrapericardially. Peribronchial lymph nodes are swept up with the mainstem bronchus and the latter is closed with a heavy wire stapler, and divided sharply. A lymph node dissection is performed for lymph nodes in the aortopulmonary, paratracheal, subcarinal, inferior pulmonary ligament, periesophageal, and any palpable locations (such as internal mammary or diaphragmatic). The bronchus can be buttressed with thymic tissue or omentum mobilized on a vascularized flap. It is preferable to avoid intercostal muscle pedicle, particularly if the rib is removed.

The diaphragm is reconstructed with a 2-mm Gore-tex patch secured to the chest wall. If an omental flap is mobilized for bronchial stump coverage, it must be advanced through a fenestration in the diaphragmatic patch.[21] A 0.1 mm lo Gore-tex or Dacron patch is fenestrated and secured in a loose, floppy fashion. The fenestrations must be large enough to prohibit tamponade but small enough not to allow herniation of the heart, in particular, of the atrial appendage. The inferior portion of the pericardial patch is secured to the diaphragmatic patch as well as the pericardial rim to prevent postoperative herniation of intraabdominal contents.

The extrapleural dissection is associated with greater fluid shifts than seen with standard pneumonectomy, in addition to a higher risk of bleeding or chylothorax. The pneumonectomy space may fill more rapidly after EPP than with standard pneumonectomy and, combined with pericardial and diaphragmatic resection/reconstruction, may lead to a more mobile mediastinum. This potential complication mandates strict management of the pneumonectomy space with many options available, including chest tube without suction, balanced drainage, intrapleural pressure monitoring, and/or intermittent aspiration of fluid/air.[29]

Extrapleural pneumonectomy postoperative care

Surgery should be performed at centers in which all members of the surgery, nursing, anesthesia, and critical care team are experienced with the postoperative management of patients undergoing EPP. Patients should be extubated to avoid positive pressure on the new bronchial stump but monitored in the intensive care unit for the early postoperative period. Prompt recognition of subtle clinical changes can prevent life-threatening complications. One such example is appropriate management of the pneumonectomy space to preclude fatal mediastinal shift.[29] Immediate identification of complications with appropriate intervention can prevent postoperative mortality.[19] Finally, careful management of fluid status and pulmonary toilet is imperative in caring for these patients postoperatively.

Most of the complications described after EPP result from injury to structures during resection. Vocal cord paralysis owing to resection and/or cautery of the recurrent laryngeal nerve can lead to poor cough and/or aspiration. If this vocal cord paresis occurs, all efforts to medialize the affected vocal cord must be made to maximize the effectiveness of pulmonary toilet. The extrapleural dissection for EPP frequently disturbs the sympathetic nerves with mild but refractory vasoplegia often seen postoperatively (frequently compounded by use of thoracic epidural anesthesia but not responsive to stopping infusion of anesthetic). This effect usually responds to oral vasoconstrictors, such as phenylephrine, which can typically be weaned in the days to weeks after surgery. Unnecessary and/or excessive fluid resuscitation in response to this benign source of hypotension should be avoided because this may precipitate right heart failure, atrial fibrillation, and/or pulmonary edema in these patients with only 1 lung remaining.

The most common complication after EPP is supraventricular arrhythmia, such as atrial fibrillation. Major morbidity, such as tamponade, cardiac or gastric herniation, patch dehiscence, myocardial infarction, chylothorax, and pulmonary embolus, occur more rarely.[13] Deep vein thrombosis is more common in MPM patients and routine screening or higher suspicion of early signs of venous thromboembolism is needed to minimize potentially fatal emboli in a patient with 1 lung. Bronchopleural fistula can occur weeks to months (and sometimes longer) after EPP and usually manifests with fever, wet cough, malaise, and an unexplained decrease in fluid level in the pneumonectomy space.

Extrapleural pneumonectomy results

Because EPP has been performed generally in the context of multimodality therapy, results reported for this operation reflect outcomes for EPP and adjuvant treatment, such as chemotherapy, radiation therapy, or immunologic therapy. In 1 series of 183 patients who underwent EPP with adjuvant chemotherapy and radiation, perioperative mortality was 3.8% and morbidity was 50% (combined major and minor complications).[2] Median survival for those who did not die perioperatively was 19 months. Epithelial cell type, negative resection margins, and lack of extrapleural nodal disease were associated with a median long-term survival of 51 months.

In a phase I study of EPP with heated intraoperative chemotherapy (HIOC), the median survival for patients who received cisplatin doses of 175 to 200 mg/m^2 was 26 months.[30] For patients with epithelial stage I or II disease, median survival was 39 months, compared with 15 months for those with stage III epithelial disease. In a larger phase II series of 121 patients who underwent EPP with HIOC, overall median survival was 12.8 months, with a median survival of 21 months for patients with early stage disease.[31]

The results of EPP and adjuvant therapy have been replicated by other groups. In a Scottish study of 302 MPM patients, those with stage I or II disease treated with EPP and adjuvant chemotherapy demonstrated a median survival of 35 months.[32] Those treated with EPP alone experienced a survival of 13 months. In a Turkish study of 20 patients undergoing EPP followed by adjuvant radiation and platinum-based chemotherapy, the median survival was 17 months.[33] Yan and colleagues[3] published a retrospective review of 70 patients undergoing EPP followed by chemotherapy and/or radiation, in which patients experienced a median survival of 20 months. Adjuvant radiation and adjuvant pemetrexed-based chemotherapy were associated independently with longer survival.

A Swiss study of 19 patients who underwent EPP after induction chemotherapy and followed by adjuvant radiation reported a median survival of 23 months, with 13 patients completing the full regimen.[5] In a large, multicenter prospective Swiss trial, the same investigators enrolled 61 patients, of whom 58 (95%) completed induction chemotherapy, 45 (74%) underwent EPP, and 36 (59%) received at least a portion of adjuvant radiotherapy.[34] Median survival was 19.8 months for all patients and 23 months for the subgroup who underwent EPP after induction chemotherapy.

Flores and associates[4] reported a phase II trial of induction chemotherapy followed by EPP followed by adjuvant hemithoracic radiation. Although the median overall survival for all patients was 19 months, the 8 patients who completed chemotherapy and EPP experienced a median survival of 35 months. A similar phase II trial involving multiple centers and cisplatin-pemetrexed instead of cisplatin-gemcitabine enrolled 77 patients, with 40 patients (52%) completing the full regimen.[35] Perioperative mortality was 3.7% and local recurrence occurred in 14% of patients. The median overall survival for all patients was 16.8 months and was 29 months for those who completed the full regimen. De Perrot and coworkers[36] published similar results in a retrospective analysis of 60 patients who underwent cisplatin-based chemotherapy followed by EPP with adjuvant hemithoracic radiation. The median survival for all patients was 14 months. Of the 30 patients (50%) who completed the full treatment regimen, those with node negative final pathology demonstrated a median survival of 59 months. The same investigators conducted a phase I/II trial enrolling 25 patients to undergo EPP within 1 week of administering 25 Gy external beam intensity-modulated radiation therapy with patients found to have mediastinal nodal disease undergoing postoperative adjuvant chemotherapy.[37] There was 1 postoperative death (4%). With a median follow-up of 23 months, the 3-year survival was 84% for patients with epithelial disease and 13% for those with nonepithelial (all biphasic) disease.

Despite advances in adjuvant therapy, local control remains the major barrier to long-term survival in MPM after EPP. Recurrence occurs in most patients, generally locoregional with rare hematogenous metastases. In the largest series to describe recurrence patterns after EPP-based multimodality therapy, Baldini and colleagues[38] reported recurrence in 75% of 158 evaluable patients (9 died perioperatively and location of recurrence not available for another 2 patients). Fifty-four patients, or 72% of all episodes of recurrence, occurred in the ipsilateral hemithorax or mediastinum as the first site. The remaining distribution of recurrence was in the abdomen (53%), contralateral chest (38%), and distant sites (7%), with many patients presenting with multiple sites of simultaneous recurrence. The authors concluded that the ipsilateral chest is the most common site of treatment failure after EPP-based multimodality therapy. Flores and colleagues[20] reported a slightly different pattern of treatment failure in a retrospective review of 663 patients undergoing surgery-based multimodality therapy on various protocols. Of 385 patients undergoing EPP, 57% experienced recurrence, with 33% of treatment failures occurring in the ipsilateral chest or pericardium as the first site of recurrence. The distribution of site of first treatment failure was abdomen (31%), contralateral chest (22%), abdomen and chest (8%), and bone (3%).

Pleurectomy Decortication

Because EPP was being scrutinized after Butchart's series suggested prohibitive mortality, there was a renewed interest in the lung-sparing P/D.[39] Many surgeons have come to recognize that macroscopic complete resection can be accomplished with less morbidity and mortality through P/D.[40]

Pleurectomy decortication preoperative evaluation

The preoperative evaluation for radical or extended P/D is identical to that for EPP. Staging, in particular, follows the procedure as outlined. The criteria for preclusive comorbidities, pulmonary function, pulmonary arterial pressures, and even ventricular function are generally considered less strict than for EPP. It is, however, sometimes difficult to predict whether P/D or EPP will be required for resection in some patients and having a thorough understanding of the patient's physiology allows for more appropriate decisions to be made intraoperatively. For example, an active elderly patient with chronic obstructive pulmonary disease, nonobstructive coronary disease, and mild left ventricular dysfunction would likely be a better candidate for P/D than for EPP, but the resectability of the tumor cannot be assessed fully until thoracotomy, and diffusely invasive disease may be found in the operating room that precludes resection by P/D. If the patient's preoperative workup suggests that EPP is prohibitive in this patient's case, resection should not be performed.

Pleurectomy decortication perioperative management

The anesthetic preparation for P/D is similar to that for EPP, particularly in light of the possibility that the plan may change from P/D to EPP. Routine lines and monitors are required. The authors do not generally use Swan-Ganz catheters for these cases and the nasogastric (or orogastric) tube is removed before extubation at the end of the case. Bleeding may be more profuse in P/D because of the decortication that comprises the visceral pleurectomy (see below) and thus large bore intravenous access is mandate, just as it is in EPP. Likewise, air leak lost through the chest tubes after visceral pleurectomy may make it difficult to inflate the lung. If the lung is expanded, even high volumes "lost" owing to air leak as reflected by lower return volumes in the bellows of the ventilator do not prohibit gas exchange in these patients because oxygenation is adequate and ventilation occurs through the ventilator and the lung surface (out the tube).

Pleurectomy decortication surgical technique

The initial approach, thoracotomy, and extrapleural dissection for P/D are similar to that of EPP, extending superiorly, inferiorly, anteriorly, and posteriorly, using the same landmarks as described. The extrapleural dissection comprises the parietal pleurectomy portion of the P/D. As the mediastinum is approached, the tumor is resected off the pericardium to the hilar cuff, if possible. If resection of the pericardium is required, it is preferable to delay the incision initiating this until a greater surface area of tumor is mobilized, because pericardial entry may precipitate arrhythmias and consequent hemodynamic instability. Likewise, the dissection of the diaphragm off the chest wall is delayed until the extent of the tumor can be assessed.

The visceral pleurectomy is equivalent to a decortication. A blade on a long handle is used to incise the tumor overlying the lung with caution not to injure the underlying lung parenchyma (a step that is easier with a bulkier tumor). A plane is developed bluntly using the Pearson scissors and Kochers are placed on the tumor to facilitate blunt dissection (using a sponge on a stick or laparotomy pad, for example) of the underlying lung parenchyma away from the tumor. The dissection is carried out, often tediously, throughout the lung surfaces, with caution in the fissures not to injure

the underlying pulmonary artery. If the diaphragm is densely involved with tumor, the lower lobe pleura/tumor is bluntly dissected off to be resected en bloc with the diaphragm. The dissection is continued inferiorly toward the inferior ligament, superiorly, anteriorly, and posteriorly to encircle the hilum.

As noted, blood loss may be substantial during P/D. Packing with laparotomy pads in areas that are not being dissected can tamponade bleeding, as can having the anesthesiologist inflate the lung (positive pressure can impede brisk bleeding). Argon beam coagulation or water-based bipolar sealants, such as Aquamantys, can be used as well. Finally, the hilum can be encircled with a red rubber catheter as a tourniquet if there is uncontrolled bleeding to allow time for coagulation, ligation, or repair of a vessel.[21] Because pneumonectomy is the "bail-out" solution to catastrophic bleeding and/or major vessel injury, the possibility of EPP must be considered in patients undergoing P/D.

As the dissection continues to the hilar cuff, the pleura thins out and it is gently peeled off the hilar structures. The specimen is frequently removed in pieces.[6] The lung can often be retracted out of bulky tumor and the inferior shell can be swept down toward the diaphragm. If the diaphragm can be preserved, even in the event of minimal residual disease, postoperative lung function and performance status is better. If there is extensive diaphragmatic invasion, resection and reconstruction are completed as described for EPP. Likewise, if the pericardium is removed owing to invasion, it is reconstructed as described. Three chest tubes are usually left to manage the pleural space, straight tubes anteriorly and posteriorly with a right angle tube over the diaphragm.

Pleurectomy decortication postoperative care

The postoperative management of P/D patients is similar to that of EPP although with less risk of pulmonary edema, right heart failure, and mediastinal shift. The remaining cardiac, pulmonary, infectious, renal, and hematologic complications that occur with EPP can also occur with P/D. The major complications unique to P/D are prolonged air leak and mucous plugging with atelectasis. Air leak is controlled with tubes, which can be placed to a Heimlich valve for more portable use. Doxycycline pleuridesis at the bedside (with tubes hung on a pole instead of clamped) has been used with limited success. Mucous plugging is frequent and prevention or treatment requires aggressive pulmonary toilet, with bronchoscopic suction if needed. One should be wary of a large air leak that disappears suddenly because this is often the result of total atelectasis of that lung and can be diagnosed on chest radiograph. In contrast, if the air leak resolves and the lung is expanded, the tube is ready for removal.

Pleurectomy decortication results

Treatment failure after P/D is most commonly found in ipsilateral chest, with 95% of sites of first recurrence occurring in the ipsilateral hemithorax and/or mediastinum in a series evaluating this question in 59 MPM patients undergoing P/D.[41] Similarly, in Flores and coworkers' series comparing EPP to P/D, 65% of first recurrences were local.[20] In an effort to decrease risk of local recurrence, various methods have been used for adjuvant therapy, just as in EPP. In a prospective phase I/II trial, 44 patients underwent P/D with HIOC, resulting in a median survival of 13 months for all resected patients and 18 months in the 35 patients who received higher doses of cisplatin HIOC (175–450 mg/m^2).[6]

Some authors have considered the remaining lung after P/D to be a limitation of adjuvant therapy in the form of external beam radiation. Several studies have demonstrated, however, that traditional hemithoracic radiation can be given safely after P/D. In the largest retrospective series of 123 patients, using a median of 42.5 Gy hemithoracic radiation after P/D, local control was seen in 42% of patients and median survival was 13.5 months.[42] The same group reported 1- and 2-year survival of 75% and 53%, respectively, using 46.8 Gy intensity-modulated radiation therapy after P/D.[43] Grade 3 or 4 pneumonitis occurred in 20% of patients.

DATA COMPARING EXTRAPLEURAL PNEUMONECTOMY WITH PLEURECTOMY DECORTICATION

P/D is associated with better short-term outcomes than EPP in the form of perioperative morbidity and mortality. One study evaluating these results in the Society of Thoracic Surgeons Database found higher rates of acute respiratory distress syndrome, reintubation, unexpected reoperation, sepsis, and mortality after EPP compared with P/D.[44]

The high risk of EPP without clear demonstration of survival benefit has led many clinicians to advocate against EPP.[45] The Mesothelioma and Radical Surgery (MARS) trial was designed to compare EPP with no surgery for MPM, but randomization was not successful in this effort. Subsequent exploratory analyses evaluating long-term outcomes lacked adequate power to draw meaningful conclusions. In the largest retrospective study comparing EPP with P/D, Flores and associates[20] concluded that the cumulative survival for patients with early stage disease was higher with curative-intent P/D compared with EPP (**Fig. 1**). For later stage disease, EPP conferred higher cumulative survival.

Several studies have sought to compare EPP with P/D. One recent metaanalysis found significantly lower mortality and a trend toward higher cumulative survival with P/D but only included a small portion of the published literature comparing the 2 operations.[23] A recent metaanalysis including all English-language observational studies from 1990 to 2014 that compared the 2 surgical procedures analyzed 24 datasets, including 1391 patients undergoing EPP and 1512 undergoing P/D (**Tables 1** and **2**).[46] The percentage of nonepithelial cases and the use and

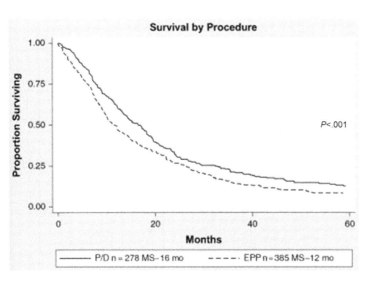

Survival by Procedure

$P<.001$

P/D n = 278 MS–16 mo   EPP n = 385 MS–12 mo

Fig. 1. Overall survival of EPP versus P/D by univariate analysis. EPP, extrapleural pneumonectomy; P/D, pleurectomy decortication. (*From* Flores RM, Pass HI, Seshan VE, et al. Extrapleural pneumonectomy versus pleurectomy/decortication in the surgical management of malignant pleural mesothelioma: results in 663 patients. J Thorac Cardiovasc Surg 2008;135:622; with permission.)

Table 1
Studies included in the metaanalysis

Author, Year	Study Design	Country	M/F	Age (y) Range, Mean ± SD	Histology	Stage	No. of P/D Patients	No. of EPP Patients	Other Treatment Before/During Surgery	Other Treatment After Surgery	Short-Term Mortality, P/D	Short-Term Mortality, EPP	Long-Term Mortality, P/D	Long-Term Mortality, EPP
Branscheid D, 1991[47]	Retro (1978–89)	Germany	235/66	22–87, median = 59	Epithelial (50%); mixed (25%); sarcomatous (12%); unclassified (13%)	I (2%); II (11%); III (56%); IV (15%)	82	76	—	Chemotherapy (49)	2.4%	11.8%	Median survival 315 d	Median survival: 284 d
Allen KB, 1994[48]	Retro (1958–93)	USA	79/17	$\mu = 55.2 \pm 1.5$ (EPP); 63.5 $\pm$ 9.6 (P)	Epithelial 56%, mixed 29%, sarcomatous 15%	I (51%); II (38%); III (8%); IV (3%)	56	40	—	73% Chemotherapy w/or w/out irradiation	3/56 (5.4%)	3/40 (7.5%)	1-, 2-, 5-y survival = 30.4%, 8.9%, 5.4%; median survival = 9 mo	1-, 2-, 5-y survival = 52.5%, 22.5%, 10%; median survival = 13.3 mo
Pass H, Kranda K, 1997[49]; Pass HI, Temeck BK, 1997[50]	Reanalysis of clinical trial (1990–95)	USA	78/17	30–77	Epithelial, 60; sarcomatoid, 6; biphasic, 12	—	39	39	Intraoperative PDT	Adjuvant chemotherapy, immunotherapy	—	—	Median survival = 14.5 mo; progression-free survival = 7.4 mo	Median survival = 9.4 mo; progression-free survival = 7 mo
Moskal TL, 1998[51]	Retro (1991–96)	USA	31/9	21–77; $\mu = 60$;	Epithelial (62.5%); biphasic (25%); sarcomatous (12.5%)	I, II = 13; III, IV = 24	28	7	—	Intracavitary PDT; palliative chemotherapy (7); radiation (7)	3.6%	28.6%	—	—
Lampi L, 1999[52]	Retro (1986–98)	Germany	45/8	n/a	Sarcomatous	II and III (PL/D)	23	22	—	—	0%	1 (4.2%)	Median survival 14 mo	Median survival 16 mo
Rusch VW, 1999[53]	Retro (1983–98)	USA	192/39	24–80; median = 62	Epithelial = 164 (71%), fibrosarcomat. = 14 (6%), Mixed = 51 (22%), demoplastic = 1, unknown = 1	I = 21; II = 40; III = 102; IV = 68	59	115	—	Radiation = 106, chemotherapy = 29; radiation + chemotherapy = 7;	0%	6/115 (5.2%)	No difference in long-term survival on multivariate analysis	—
Aziz T, 2002[54]	Retro (1989–99)	UK	244/61	34–77; median = 57	Epithelial and sarcomatous	I, II, III	47	64	—	Intrapleural and systemic chemotherapy	0%	6/64 (9.1%)	Median survival = 14 mo	Median survival = 13 mo; with chemotherapy double survival vs no chemotherapy
Yom SS, 2003[55]	Phase I trial on PDT	UK	8/1	39–75	Epithelioid = 7, biphasic = 2	—	8	1	—	PDT	—	—	2/7 died at 14 mo	All alive at 14 mo

Study	Design (years)	Country	M/F	Age	Histology	Stage	n	n	Treatment	Treatment detail	%	%	Survival	Survival
de Vries WI, 2003[56]	Retro (1976–2001)	South Africa	33/13	35–80	Epithelial, sarcomatoid, mixed	I, II, III	29	17	—	Chemotherapy and radiation (23); chemotherapy (13); radiation (3); no chemotherapy or radiation (5)	3.8%	5.8%	Median survival = 9 mo	Median survival = 12 mo
Rosenzweig KE, 2005[57]	Phase II trial (1994–1996)	USA	—	—	—	T2 - T3, N0-N2	6	7	IORT	External beam radiation therapy (n = 9)	1/6	1/7	2-y actuarial overall survival = 33%	2-y actuarial overall survival = 14%
Flores RM, 2007[58]	Retro (1990–2005)	USA	755/190	26–93; median = 66	Epithelioid = 319 (34%), mixed = 99 (10%), sarcomatoid = 44 (5%), unclassified = 483 (51%)	I (2%); II (95%); III (24%); IV (16%), unknown (48%)	176	208	—	Radiation = 130, chemotherapy = 35, chemotherapy + radiation = 42	5 (3%)	11 (5%)	Median survival = 15.8 mo	Median survival = 14.3 mo
Okada M, 2008[59]	Retro (1986–2006)	Japan	58/7	35–78; median = 60 y	Epithelial (74%), mixed (17%), sarcomatous (9%)	I (12%), II (20%), III (62%), IV (6%)	34	31	—	Chemotherapy and radiotherapy	0%	3.2%	3-y survival = 24%; median survival = 17 mo	3-y survival = 33%; median survival = 13 mo
Schipper PH, 2008[60]	Retro (1985–2003)	USA	236/49	26–91; median 66	Epithelial = 134, nonepithelial = 108, unclassified = 43	IA = 20, IB = 82, II = 24, III = 75, IV = 60, unknown = 24	44	73	Chemotherapy = 9 (2%); combination of chemotherapy and radiation = 18 (6%)	Chemotherapy = 42 (15%), radiotherapy = 16 (6%), combination = 24 (8%)	1 (2.9%)	6 (8.2%)	1-, 2-y survival = 80% and 35%; 30%, 15% (subtotal P/D)	1-, 2-y survival l = 61%, 25%;
Borasio P, 2008[61]	Retro (1989–2003)	Italy	270/124	28–93; median = 64	Epithelial = 246 (67.2%), biphasic = 84 (23%), sarcomatous = 36 (9.8%), indeterminate = 28	—	12	15	—	Multimodal therapy, chemotherapy (P/D), chemotherapy (EPP)	Morbidity = 4	Mortality = 1; morbidity = 9	Mortality = 1;	—
Yan TD, 2009[62]	Retro (1984–2007)	Australia	390/66	66 ± 10	Epithelial = 185 (40%), sarcomatoid/biphasic = 183 (40%), unknown = 88 (19%)	×	250	59	Combination chemotherapy	Radiotherapy = 40 (9%), combination chemotherapy = 45 (10%)	—	4	18-mo survival = 63, 25%	18-mo survival = 30, 51%
Mineo TC, 2010[63]	Retro (1987–2007)	Italy	63/14	27–82; 61.3 ± 10	Epithelioid = 50, biphasic = 17, sarcomatoid = 10	I = 21, II = 3 6, III = 20	44 (10 subtotal)	27	Neoadjuvant from 2006	Radiotherapy = 17, radiochemotherapy = 56, neoadjuvant chemotherapy plus radiotherapy = 4	0	1	Major morbidity rate = 6/44, 14%; median survival = 10 mo	Major morbidity rate = 9/27, 33%; median survival = 11 mo
Luckraz H, 2010[64]	Retro (1980–2010)	UK	180/28	58.9 ± 9.8	Epithelial	I, II, III	90	49	Chemotherapy and radiation	Chemotherapy = 13 (P/D), 14 (EPP); radio = 19 (P/D), 8 (EPP); chemotherapy and radio = 24 (P/D) + 15 (EPP)	1.1%	8.2%	2-y survival = 9%; median survival = 8.3 mo	2-y survival = 8%; median survival = 3.3 mo

(continued on next page)

Table 1
(continued)

Author, Year	Study Design	Country	M/F	Age (y) Range, Mean ± SD	Histology	Stage	No. of P/D Patients	No. of EPP Patients	Other Treatment Before/During Surgery	Other Treatment After Surgery	Short-Term Mortality, P/D	Short-Term Mortality, EPP	Long-Term Mortality, P/D	Long-Term Mortality, EPP
Friedberg JS, 2011[65]	Retro (2004–08)	USA	19/9	27–81	Epithelioid n = 17, sarcomatoid = 2, biphasic = 3	III, IV (85.7%)	14	14	Chemotherapy (n = 4, EPP; n = 2 PL)	Chemotherapy (n = 9, P/D; n = 7, EPP); radiotherapy (n = 6, P/D; n = 9, EPP)- PDT	0	2	Median survival = not reached; median disease-free survival = 1.9 y	Median survival = 0.7 y; median disease-free survival = 0.6 y
Rena O, 2012[66]	Retro (1998–2009)	Italy	24/35	56 ± 11 (EPP); 58.5 ± 9.5 (P/D)	Epithelial = 29	I, II	37	40	Neoadjuvant	Chemotherapy	—	—	Recurrence rate = 56%; median survival after recurrence = 14 mo	Recurrence rate = 21%; median survival after recurrence = 9 mo EPP
Nakas A, Waller D, 2012[67]; Nakas A, Meyenfeldt E, 2012[68]; [Martin-Ucar AE, 2007[69]]	Retro	UK	181/31	14–72; median = 59	Epithelioid = 160, biphasic = 52	×	85	127	Chemotherapy (n = 25, EPP and n = 8, PL)	Chemotherapy (n = 32/53 [P/D]; 26/71 [EPP]); radical hemithorax irradiation (n = 33/98)	3%	7%	2-, 3-, 5-y survival = 31.6%, 16.8%, 4.8%; median survival = 13.4 mo; 90 d mortality = 8 (12%)	2-, 3-, 5-y survival = 34.4%, 17.3%, 8%; median survival = 15.6 mo; 90 d mortality = 17 (17%)

Study	Design (period)	Country	n (P/D / EPP)	Age	Histology	Stage	n (P/D)	n (EPP)	Neoadjuvant	Other therapy	Mortality (P/D)	Mortality (EPP)	Survival (P/D)	Survival (EPP)
Lang-Lazdunski L, 2012[70]	Retro (2004–2011)	UK	x	x	Epithelioid and nonepitheliod	I–IV	61	25	Neoadjuvant	17 = radiotherapy (EPP); radiotherapy + chemotherapy = 54 (P/D)	0%	4.5%	2-y survival = 49%; 5-y = 30.1%; median survival = 23 mo	2-y survival = 18.2%; 5-y = 9%; median survival = 12.8 mo
Lindenmann J, 2012[71]	Retro (2000–2009)	Austria	47/14	34–82; mean = 63.7	Epithelioid = 48 (78.7%), sarcomatoid = 3 (4.9%), biphasic = 10 (16%)	—	41	3	PDT	Chemotherapy, pleurodesis	0	0	Similar survival (not shown)	
Bedirhan MA, 2013[72]	Retro (2001–13)	Turkey	58/18	30–76 (mean 53.2)	Epithelioid = 60	—	45	31	—	Adjuvant chemotherapy	0%; 1 (4%) E/P	4 (12.9%)	Median survival = 15-mo; 3-y survival = 13%; 5-y = 0%. (E/P: median survival 27 mo; 3 y 34%)	Median survival 17-mo; 3-y = 21%; 5-y = 17%
Bovolato P, 2014[73]	Retro (1982–2012)	Italy	374/129	62.5 (P/D); 58.7 (EPP)	Epithelial 81%	I: 9.5%, II: 27.6%; >/= III: 19%; unknown: 43.7%	202	301	—	—	2.6%	4.1%	Median survival = 20.5 mo; 2- and 5-y survival = 40% and 10%	Median survival 18.8 mo; 2- and 5-y survival = 37% and 12%

Abbreviations: EPP, extrapleural pneumonectomy; IORT, intraoperative radiotherapy; n/a, not applicable; P/D, pleurectomy/decortication; PDT, photodynamic therapy.

From Taioli ET, Wolf AS, Flores RM. Meta-analysis of survival after pleurectomy decortication versus extrapleural pneumonectomy in mesothelioma. Ann Thorac Surg 2015;99:473; with permission.

Table 2
Complications after P/D and EPP

Author, Year	Number of Cases P/D, EPP	Complications P/D	Complications EPP
Allen, 1994[48]	56, 40	26.8% (15 cases) prolonged air leakage (6), arrhythmias (5), tracheostomy (2), renal failure (2), pneumonia (1)	30% (12 cases); bronchopleural fistula (2), vocal cord paralysis (2), arrhythmias (3), tracheostomy (2), chylothorax (1), MI (1) contralateral benign pleural effusion (1), splenectomy (1), pneumonia (1)
Pass, Kranda, 1997[49]; Pass, Temeck, 1997[50]	39, 39	Supraventricular tachyarrhythmias (2), postoperative pancreatitis (4), esophageal-pleural fistula (2), hemorrhage (2), diaphragmatic herniation (1), temporary left radial nerve palsy (1), wound dehiscence (1)[a]	Supraventricular tachyarrhythmias (14), bronchopleural fistulae (7)
Aziz, 2002[54]	47, 64	Reexploration for bleeding (1), pneumonia (1)	21% (14 cases); ARDS (6), pneumonia (4), bleeding (4), reintubation and ventilation (2)
de Vries, 2003[56]	29, 17	Empyema (1)	Atelectasis (2), prolonged air leak (3), discharge with drainage (1), prolonged ventilation (1), large blood transfusion (3)
Rosenzweig, 2005[57]	6, 7	Pneumonitis/transesophageal fistula (1), chest tube leak (1)	Thoracic duct leak (1), empyema (1), wound dehiscence (1)
Okada, 2008[59]	34, 31	15%; supraventricular arrhythmias (3), respiratory infection (2),	48%; supraventricular arrhythmias (8), respiratory failure (4), respiratory infection (1), bleeding (2), heart hernia (2), bronchial stump insufficiency (2), chylothorax (2), heart failure (1), laryngeal nerve palsy (1)
Schipper, 2008[60]	44, 73	4 (9%) bleeding, respiratory failure (1), MI (1)	37 (50.5%); empyema (14), respiratory failure (10), bronchopleural fistulae, bleeding (5), orthostatic hypotension (5), ARDS (4), bowel herniation (4), MI (3), acute renal failure (3), cerebrovascular accident (3), pulmonary embolism (3), cardiac herniation (2), vocal cord paralysis (2), gastric perforation (1), heart failure (1), pleurocutaneous fistulae (1), splenic rupture (1), esophageal perforation (1), delayed gastric emptying (1), metabolic encephalopathy (1), gastropleural fistula (1)
Borasio, 2008[61]	12, 15	33% (4 cases); Bleeding (2), atrial fibrillation (1), retained secretions (1)	60% (9 cases); atrial fibrillation (4), respiratory failure (3), bleeding (3), ileus (2), pneumonia (1), vocal cord paralysis (1)

Mineo, 2010[63]	44, 27	13.6% (6 cases); bleeding (4), DVT (2)	33% (9 cases); cardiac arrhythmias (4), bleeding (2), vocal cord palsy (1), DVT (2), bronchopleural fistula (2)
Luckraz, 2010[64]	90, 49	Atrial fibrillation (8)	Infections (8), bronchopleural fistula (7), atrial fibrillation (2)
Friedberg, 2011[65]	14,14	DVT requiring anticoagulation (4) atrial fibrillation (3), chyle leak (2), pneumonia (3), respiratory failure (1), persistent air leak (1)	DVT requiring anticoagulation (6) atrial fibrillation (3), chyle leak (1), pneumonia (2), Respiratory failure (2), pulmonary embolism (1), stroke (1), MI (1)
Rena, 2012[66]	37, 40	24% (9 cases); atrial fibrillation (2), bleeding requiring operation (1), MI (1)	62% (25 cases); atrial fibrillation (17), bleeding requiring operation (2), pneumonia (2), ARDS (1), cerebral ischemic attack (1), pulmonary embolism (1), bronchopleural fistula with empyema (1), gastric hernia after diaphragmatic prosthesis dislocation (1)
Nakas, Waller, 2012[67]; Nakas, Meyenfeldt, 2012[68]	85, 127	Reoperation (5), prolonged air leak (20), pleural sepsis (5)	Reoperation (19), pleural sepsis (8)
Lang-Lazdunski, 2012[70]	61, 25	27.7%; Arrhythmia (2), persistent air leak (10), chylothorax (4) ARDS (1)	68%; Arrhythmia (7), reoperation for bleeding (2), bronchopleural fistula/empyema (2), pulmonary embolus (1), ARDS (1), pneumonia (1), vocal cord palsy (1), Horner's syndrome (1), late septicemia (1)
Bovolato, 2014[73]	202, 301	21.6% (65 cases); atrial fibrillation (32), bleeding (13), chest infection (4), bronchopleural fistula (3), pulmonary embolism, (3), displacement of diaphragmatic prosthesis with herniation (3), respiratory insufficiency (2), DVT (2), ARDS (1), cerebral ischemia (1), wound infection (1)	10.4% (21 cases); atrial fibrillation (9), prolonged air leak (5), bleeding (3); MI (2), contralateral pleural effusion (1), paraplegia (1)

Abbreviations: ARDS, acute respiratory distress syndrome; DVT, deep venous thrombosis; MI, myocardial infarction.

a These complications are reported in general, not assigned to one or the other surgical procedure.

From Taioli ET, Wolf AS, Flores RM. Meta-analysis of survival after pleurectomy decortication versus extrapleural pneumonectomy in mesothelioma. Ann Thorac Surg 2015;99:478; with permission.

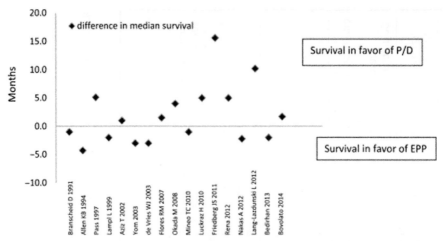

Fig. 2. Difference in median survival between pleurectomy decortications (P/D) and extrapleural pneumonectomy (EPP; number of studies = 17). (*From* Taioli ET, Wolf AS, Flores RM. Meta-analysis of survival after pleurectomy decortication versus extrapleural pneumonectomy in mesothelioma. Ann Thorac Surg 2015;99:476; with permission.)

types of adjuvant treatment varied from study to study. There was significantly higher 30-day mortality associated with EPP (4.5% vs 1.7%; $P<.05$) with little heterogeneity between studies. Among the 17 studies that reported median survival, 53% reported higher median survival with EPP (and 47% with P/D). Of the 7 studies reporting at least 2-year survival, survival was similar for the cohorts, but there was significant heterogeneity among studies (**Fig. 2**).[46]

SUMMARY

Despite decades of application in practice, the role of surgery in the treatment of MPM is not considered standard and there is certainly no procedure of choice. Although it does not seem that a randomized trial can be done to shed light on this issue, the evidence is clear that P/D is better tolerated by patients and suggests that survival is no worse. Because recurrence patterns are generally local regardless of operation, leaving the patient with 2 lungs after first surgery may well improve the ability to tolerate further therapy, and may explain the trend toward longer survival seen with P/D. Without a substantial benefit in terms of long-term outcomes, the added risk of EPP may not be worth assuming for most MPM patients. Although EPP is still performed in certain cases, the authors advocate radical P/D whenever possible for patients with MPM.

REFERENCES

1. Taioli E, Wolf AS, Moline JM, et al. Frequency of surgery in black patients with malignant pleural mesothelioma. Dis Markers 2015;2015:282145.

2. Sugarbaker DJ, Flores RM, Jaklitsch MT, et al. Resection margins, extrapleural nodal status, and cell type determine postoperative long-term survival in trimodality therapy of malignant pleural mesothelioma: results in 183 patients. J Thorac Cardiovasc Surg 1999;117(1):54–63 [discussion: 63–5].

3. Yan TD, Boyer M, Tin MM, et al. Extrapleural pneumonectomy for malignant pleural mesothelioma: outcomes of treatment and prognostic factors. J Thorac Cardiovasc Surg 2009;138(3):619–24.

4. Flores RM, Krug LM, Rosenzweig KE, et al. Induction chemotherapy, extrapleural pneumonectomy, and postoperative high-dose radiotherapy for locally advanced malignant pleural mesothelioma: a phase II trial. J Thorac Oncol 2006;1(4):289–95.

5. Weder W, Kestenholz P, Taverna C, et al. Neoadjuvant chemotherapy followed by extrapleural pneumonectomy in malignant pleural mesothelioma. J Clin Oncol 2004;22(17):3451–7.

6. Richards WG, Zellos L, Bueno R, et al. Phase I to II study of pleurectomy/decortication and intraoperative intracavitary hyperthermic cisplatin lavage for mesothelioma. J Clin Oncol 2006; 24(10):1561–7.

7. Pass HI, Temeck BK, Kranda K, et al. Phase III randomized trial of surgery with or without intraoperative photodynamic therapy and postoperative immunochemotherapy for malignant pleural mesothelioma. Ann Surg Oncol 1997;4(8):628–33.

8. de Perrot M, Feld R, Leighl NB, et al. Accelerated hemithoracic radiation followed by extrapleural pneumonectomy for malignant pleural mesothelioma. J Thorac Cardiovasc Surg 2016;151(2):468–75.

9. Kindler HL, Karrison TG, Gandara DR, et al. Multicenter, double-blind, placebo-controlled, randomized phase II trial of gemcitabine/cisplatin plus

bevacizumab or placebo in patients with malignant mesothelioma. J Clin Oncol 2012;30(20):2509–15.

10. Wolf AS, Richards WG, Tilleman TR, et al. Characteristics of malignant pleural mesothelioma in in women. Ann Thorac Surg 2010;90(3):949–56 [discussion: 95].

11. Sugarbaker DJ, Wolf AS. Surgery for malignant pleural mesothelioma. Expert Rev Respir Med 2010;4(3):363–72.

12. Taioli E, Wolf AS, Camacho-Rivera M, et al. Women with malignant pleural mesothelioma have a three-fold better survival rate than men. Ann Thorac Surg 2014;98(3):1020–4.

13. Sugarbaker DJ, Wolf AS, Chirieac LR, et al. Clinical and pathological features of three-year survivors of malignant pleural mesothelioma following extrapleural pneumonectomy. Eur J Cardiothorac Surg 2011; 40(2):298–303.

14. Chirieac LR, Corson JM. Pathologic evaluation of malignant pleural mesothelioma. Semin Thorac Cardiovasc Surg 2009;21(2):121–4.

15. Flores RM, Riedel E, Donington JS, et al. Frequency of use and predictors of cancer-directed surgery in the management of malignant pleural mesothelioma in a community-based (Surveillance, Epidemiology, and End Results [SEER]) population. J Thorac Oncol 2010;5(10):1649–54.

16. Flores RM, Zakowski M, Venkatraman E, et al. Prognostic factors in the treatment of malignant pleural mesothelioma at a large tertiary referral center. J Thorac Oncol 2007;2(10):957–65.

17. Sarot IA. Extrapleural pneumonectomy and pleurectomy in pulmonary tuberculosis. Thorax 1949;4(4): 173–223.

18. Butchart EG, Ashcroft T, Barnsley WC, et al. Pleuropneumonectomy in the management of diffuse malignant mesothelioma of the pleura. Experience with 29 patients. Thorax 1976;31(1): 15–24.

19. Sugarbaker DJ, Jaklitsch MT, Bueno R, et al. Prevention, early detection, and management of complications after 328 consecutive extrapleural pneumonectomies. J Thorac Cardiovasc Surg 2004;128(1):138–46.

20. Flores RM, Pass HI, Seshan VE, et al. Extrapleural pneumonectomy versus pleurectomy/decortication in the surgical management of malignant pleural mesothelioma: results in 663 patients. J Thorac Cardiovasc Surg 2008; 135(3):620–6.e1-3.

21. Wolf AS, Daniel J, Sugarbaker DJ. Surgical techniques for multimodality treatment of malignant pleural mesothelioma: extrapleural pneumonectomy and pleurectomy/decortication. Semin Thorac Cardiovasc Surg 2009;21(2):132–48.

22. Flores RM. Surgical options in malignant pleural mesothelioma: extrapleural pneumonectomy or pleurectomy/decortication. Semin Thorac Cardiovasc Surg 2009;21(2):149–53.

23. Cao C, Tian D, Park J, et al. A systematic review and meta-analysis of surgical treatments for malignant pleural mesothelioma. Lung Cancer 2014;83(2): 240–5.

24. Flores RM. The role of PET in the surgical management of malignant pleural mesothelioma. Lung Cancer 2005;49(Suppl 1):S27–32.

25. Flores RM, Routledge T, Seshan VE, et al. The impact of lymph node station on survival in 348 patients with surgically resected malignant pleural mesothelioma: implications for revision of the American Joint Committee on cancer staging system. J Thorac Cardiovasc Surg 2008;136(3):605–10.

26. Sugarbaker DJ, Richards WG, Bueno R. Extrapleural pneumonectomy in the treatment of epithelioid malignant pleural mesothelioma: novel prognostic implications of combined N1 and N2 nodal involvement based on experience in 529 patients. Ann Surg 2014;260(4):577–80 [discussion: 580–2].

27. Patz EF Jr, Shaffer K, Piwnica-Worms DR, et al. Malignant pleural mesothelioma: value of CT and MR imaging in predicting resectability. AJR Am J Roentgenol 1992;159(5):961–6.

28. Ng JM, Hartigan PM. Anesthetic management of patients undergoing extrapleural pneumonectomy for mesothelioma. Curr Opin Anaesthesiol 2008;21(1): 21–7.

29. Wolf AS, Jacobson FL, Tilleman TR, et al. Managing the pneumonectomy space after extrapleural pneumonectomy: postoperative intrathoracic pressure monitoring. Eur J Cardiothorac Surg 2010;37(4): 770–5.

30. Sugarbaker DJ, Gill RR, Yeap BY, et al. Hyperthermic intraoperative pleural cisplatin chemotherapy extends interval to recurrence and survival among low-risk patients with malignant pleural mesothelioma undergoing surgical macroscopic complete resection. J Thorac Cardiovasc Surg 2013;145(4): 955–63.

31. Tilleman TR, Richards WG, Zellos L, et al. Extrapleural pneumonectomy followed by intracavitary intraoperative hyperthermic cisplatin with pharmacologic cytoprotection for treatment of malignant pleural mesothelioma: a phase II prospective study. J Thorac Cardiovasc Surg 2009;138(2):405–11.

32. Aziz T, Jilaihawi A, Prakash D. The management of malignant pleural mesothelioma; single centre experience in 10 years. Eur J Cardiothorac Surg 2002; 22(2):298–305.

33. Batirel HF, Metintas M, Caglar HB, et al. Trimodality treatment of malignant pleural mesothelioma. J Thorac Oncol 2008;3(5):499–504.

34. Weder W, Stahel RA, Bernhard J, et al. Multicenter trial of neo-adjuvant chemotherapy followed by

extrapleural pneumonectomy in malignant pleural mesothelioma. Ann Oncol 2007;18(7):1196–202.

35. Krug LM, Pass HI, Rusch VW, et al. Multicenter phase II trial of neoadjuvant pemetrexed plus cisplatin followed by extrapleural pneumonectomy and radiation for malignant pleural mesothelioma. J Clin Oncol 2009;27(18):3007–13.

36. de Perrot M, Feld R, Cho BC, et al. Trimodality therapy with induction chemotherapy followed by extrapleural pneumonectomy and adjuvant high-dose hemithoracic radiation for malignant pleural mesothelioma. J Clin Oncol 2009;27(9):1413–8.

37. Cho BC, Feld R, Leighl N, et al. A feasibility study evaluating surgery for mesothelioma after radiation therapy: the "SMART" approach for resectable malignant pleural mesothelioma. J Thorac Oncol 2014;9(3):397–402.

38. Baldini EH, Richards WG, Gill RR, et al. Updated patterns of failure after multimodality therapy for malignant pleural mesothelioma. J Thorac Cardiovasc Surg 2015;149(5):1374–81.

39. McCormack PM, Nagasaki F, Hilaris BS, et al. Surgical treatment of pleural mesothelioma. J Thorac Cardiovasc Surg 1982;84(6):834–42.

40. Flores RM. Pleurectomy decortication for mesothelioma: the procedure of choice when possible. J Thorac Cardiovasc Surg 2016;151(2):310–2.

41. Wolf AS, Gill RR, Baldini EH, et al. Patterns of recurrence following pleurectomy/decortication for malignant pleural mesothelioma. In: 11th International Conference of the International Mesothelioma Interest Group. Boston, December 28, 2012.

42. Gupta V, Mychalczak B, Krug L, et al. Hemithoracic radiation therapy after pleurectomy/decortication for malignant pleural mesothelioma. Int J Radiat Oncol Biol Phys 2005;63(4):1045–52.

43. Rosenzweig KE, Zauderer MG, Laser B, et al. Pleural intensity-modulated radiotherapy for malignant pleural mesothelioma. Int J Radiat Oncol Biol Phys 2012;83(4):1278–83.

44. Burt BM, Cameron RB, Mollberg NM, et al. Malignant pleural mesothelioma and the society of thoracic surgeons database: an analysis of surgical morbidity and mortality. J Thorac Cardiovasc Surg 2014;148(1):30–5.

45. Treasure T, Lang-Lazdunski L, Waller D, et al. Extra-pleural pneumonectomy versus no extrapleural pneumonectomy for patients with malignant pleural mesothelioma: clinical outcomes of the Mesothelioma and Radical Surgery (MARS) randomised feasibility study. Lancet Oncol 2011;12(8):763–72.

46. Taioli E, Wolf AS, Flores RM. Meta-analysis of survival after pleurectomy decortication versus extrapleural pneumonectomy in mesothelioma. Ann Thorac Surg 2015;99(2):472–80.

47. Branscheid D, Krysa S, Bauer E, et al. Diagnostic and therapeutic strategy in malignant pleural mesothelioma. Eur J Cardiothorac Surg 1991;5:466–72.

48. Allen KB, Faber LP, Warren WH. Malignant pleural mesothelioma. Extrapleural pneumonectomy and pleurectomy. Chest Surg Clin N Am 1994;4:113–26.

49. Pass HI, Kranda K, Temeck BK, et al. Surgically debulked malignant pleural mesothelioma: results and prognostic factors. Ann Surg Oncol 1997;4:215–22.

50. Pass HI, Temeck BK, Kranda K, et al. Phase III randomized trial of surgery with or without intraoperative photodynamic therapy and postoperative immunochemotherapy for malignant pleural mesothelioma. Ann Surg Oncol 1997;4:628–33.

51. Moskal TL, Dougherty TJ, Urschel JD, et al. Operation and photodynamic therapy for pleural mesothelioma: 6-year follow-up. Ann Thorac Surg 1998;66:1128–33.

52. Lampl L, Jakob R. How should we treat malignant pleural mesothelioma (MPM)? Acta Chir Hung 1999;38:87–90.

53. Rusch VW, Venkatraman ES. Important prognostic factors in patients with malignant pleural mesothelioma, managed surgically. Ann Thorac Surg 1999;68:1799–804.

54. Aziz T, Jilaihawi A, Prakash D. The management of malignant pleural mesothelioma; single centre experience in 10 years. Eur J Cardiothorac Surg 2002;22:298–305.

55. Yom SS, Busch TM, Friedberg JS, et al. Elevated serum cytokine levels in mesothelioma patients who have undergone pleurectomy or extrapleural pneumonectomy and adjuvant intraoperative photodynamic therapy. Photochem Photobiol 2003;78:75–81.

56. de Vries WJ, Long MA. Treatment of mesothelioma in Bloemfontein, South Africa. Eur J Cardiothorac Surg 2003;24:434–40.

57. Rosenzweig KE, Fox JL, Zelefsky MJ, et al. A pilot trial of high-dose-rate intraoperative radiation therapy for malignant pleural mesothelioma. Brachytherapy 2005;4:30–3.

58. Flores RM, Zakowski M, Venkatraman E, et al. Prognostic factors in the treatment of malignant pleural mesothelioma at a large tertiary referral center. J Thorac Oncol 2007;2:957–65.

59. Okada M, Mimura T, Ohbayashi C, et al. Radical surgery for malignant pleural mesothelioma: results and prognosis. Interact Cardiovasc Thorac Surg 2008;7:102–6.

60. Schipper PH, Nichols FC, Thomse KM, et al. Malignant pleural mesothelioma: surgical management in 285 patients. Ann Thorac Surg 2008;85:257–64.

61. Borasio P, Berruti A, Billé A, et al. Malignant pleural mesothelioma: clinicopathologic and survival characteristics in a consecutive series of 394 patients. Eur J Cardiothorac Surg 2008;33:307–13.

62. Yan TD, Boyer M, Tin MM, et al. Prognostic features of long-term survivors after surgical management of malignant pleural mesothelioma. Ann Thorac Surg 2009;87:1552–6.

63. Mineo TC, Ambrogi V, Cufari ME, et al. May cyclooxygenase-2 (COX-2), p21 and p27 expression affect prognosis and therapeutic strategy of patients with malignant pleural mesothelioma? Eur J Cardiothorac Surg 2010;38:245–52.

64. Luckraz H, Rahman M, Patel N, et al. Three decades of experience in the surgical multi-modality management of pleural mesothelioma. Eur J Cardiothorac Surg 2010;37:552–6.

65. Friedberg JS, Mick R, Culligan M, et al. Photodynamic therapy and the evolution of a lung-sparing surgical treatment for mesothelioma. Ann Thorac Surg 2011;91:1738–45.

66. Rena O, Casadio C. Extrapleural pneumonectomy for early stage malignant pleural mesothelioma: a harmful procedure. Lung Cancer 2012;77:151–5.

67. Nakas A, Waller D, Lau K, et al. The new case for cervical mediastinoscopy in selection for radical surgery for malignant pleural mesothelioma. Eur J Cardiothorac Surg 2012;42:72–6.

68. Nakas A, von Meyenfeldt E, Lau K, et al. Long-term survival after lung-sparing total pleurectomy for locally advanced (International Mesothelioma Interest Group Stage T3-T4) non-sarcomatoid malignant pleural mesothelioma. Eur J Cardiothorac Surg 2012;41:1031–6.

69. Martin-Ucar AE, Nakas A, Edwards JG, et al. Case-control study between extrapleural pneumonectomy and radical pleurectomy/decortication for pathological N2 malignant pleural mesothelioma. Eur J Cardiothorac Surg 2007;31:765–70.

70. Lang-Lazdunski L, Bille A, Lal R, et al. Pleurectomy/decortication is superior to extrapleural pneumonectomy in the multimodality management of patients with malignant pleural mesothelioma. J Thorac Oncol 2012;7:737–43.

71. Lindenmann J, Matzi V, Neuboeck N, Anegg U, et al. Multimodal therapy of malignant pleural mesothelioma: is the replacement of radical surgery imminent? Interact Cardiovasc Thorac Surg 2013;16:237–43.

72. Bedirhan MA, Cansever L, Demir A, et al. Which type of surgery should become the preferred procedure for malignant pleural mesothelioma: extrapleural pneumonectomy or extended pleurectomy? J Thorac Dis 2013;5:446–54.

73. Bovolato P, Casadio C, Billè A, et al. Does surgery improve survival of patients with malignant pleural mesothelioma?: a multicenter retrospective analysis of 1365 consecutive patients. J Thorac Oncol 2014;9:390–6.

Index

Note: Page numbers of article titles are in **boldface** type.

A

Adenocarcinoma
   and sublobar resection, 254, 257
Adjuvant chemotherapy
   and evaluation in major studies, 278
   in patients who have received neoadjuvant
      chemotherapy, 278, 279
   survival benefit of, 278
Adrenal metastases
   and oligometastatic non–small cell lung cancer,
      290, 291
Axillary hiperhidrosis
   and video-assisted thoracic sympathectomy,
      349, 352

B

Best approach and benefit of plication for paralyzed
   diaphragm, **333–346**
Brain metastases
   and oligometastatic non–small cell lung cancer,
      289, 290
Breast carcinoma
   and lymph node metastasis, 319, 320
   and pulmonary metastasis, 319, 320

C

Colorectal carcinoma
   and lymph node metastasis, 316, 317
   and pulmonary metastasis, 316, 317
Controlled pneumothorax
   and diaphragmatic plication, 340
Cranial-facial hiperhidrosis
   and video-assisted thoracic sympathectomy,
      349, 352
Current treatment of mesothelioma: Extrapleural
   pneumonectomy versus pleurectomy/
   decortication, **359–375**

D

Diaphragmatic paralysis
   and chest radiography, 335
   clinical presentation of, 334
   and computed tomography, 335
   diagnosis of, 334, 335
   and diaphragmatic eventration, 333
   and diaphragmatic plication, 335, 336
   and fluoroscopic sniff test, 335
   and imaging studies, 335
   and magnetic resonance imaging, 335
   pathophysiology of, 334
   and physical evaluation, 334
   and preoperative evaluation, 334, 335
   and pulmonary function tests, 334, 335
   and quality of life evaluation, 334
   and respiratory evaluation, 334
   surgical treatment for, 335–344
   and symptom evaluation, 334
   and ultrasonography, 335
Diaphragmatic plication
   anesthesia for, 338
   and anterior plication, 340–342
   and clinical results in the literature, 343
   comparison of surgical approaches for, 344
   complications of, 342–344
   contraindications to, 336
   and controlled pneumothorax, 340
   and exposure, 340
   indications for, 336
   laparoscopic, 338
   and lung reexpansion, 342
   open transabdominal, 337
   open transthoracic, 336, 337
   patient positioning for, 338, 339
   ports for, 340
   and posterior plication, 340
   and postoperative care, 342
   procedure steps for, 340–342
   and rehabilitation and recovery, 344
   robotic-assisted, 337
   surgical approaches for, 336–338
   suture material for, 340
   technique for, 338–342
   and tube thoracostomy, 342
   and video-assisted thoracoscopic surgery, 337

E

EBUS-EUS. See *Endobronchial
   ultrasound–endoscopic ultrasound.*
Endobronchial ultrasound–endoscopic ultrasound
   accuracy of, 244–246
   and aortopulmonary window lymph nodes, 247
   complication rate for, 246, 247
   cost of, 247
   and lymph node access, 244–246

Thorac Surg Clin 26 (2016) 377–381
http://dx.doi.org/10.1016/S1547-4127(16)30037-8
1547-4127/16/$ – see front matter

Endobronchial (*continued*)
    and mediastinal staging, 244–247
    and negative predictive value, 244–246
    and restaging after chemoradiation, 247
    sensitivity of, 244–246
EPP. See *Extrapleural pneumonectomy.*
Esophageal cancer
    and esophagectomy, 295, 296, 300, 301
    and induction chemoradiation, 299, 300
    and induction chemotherapy, 298, 299
    induction chemotherapy vs. induction
        chemoradiation, 300, 301
    induction therapy for, 295–301
    and selection of induction therapy, 301
    staging of, 296, 297
Esophageal perforation
    and stent placement, 305–313
Esophagectomy
    for esophageal cancer, 295, 296, 300, 301
The evolution and current utility of esophageal stent
    placement for the treatment of acute esophageal
    perforation, **305–314**
Extrapleural pneumonectomy
    complications after, 370
    for malignant pleural mesothelioma, 360–363
    and perioperative management, 361
    and postoperative care, 362
    preoperative evaluation for, 360, 361
    results of, 362, 363
    surgical technique for, 361, 362
    vs. pleurectomy/decortication, 365–372

G

Germ cell tumors
    and lymph node metastasis, 318, 319
    and pulmonary metastasis, 318, 319
GGN. See *Ground glass nodules.*
Ground glass nodules
    and sublobar resection, 257

H

Hiperhidrosis
    axillary, 349, 352
    cranial-facial, 349, 352
    oxibutinin for, 353
    palmar, 348, 351, 352
    plantar, 348, 349, 352
    and quality of life, 353, 354
    video-assisted thoracic sympathectomy for,
        347–357
Horner syndrome
    and video-assisted thoracic sympathectomy, 356
Hybrid treatment strategy

    and stent placement for esophageal perforation,
        306, 307, 312
Hyperhidrosis
    and video-assisted thoracic sympathectomy,
        347–357

I

Immunotherapy
    and non–small cell lung cancer, 281
Induction chemoradiation
    and randomized trials of esophageal cancer
        patients, 299
    and thymoma, 328–330
Induction chemotherapy
    and randomized trials of esophageal cancer
        patients, 298
    and thymoma, 326–328
Induction radiation
    and thymoma, 330
Induction therapy
    benefits of, 331
Induction therapy for thymoma, **325–332**
Intergroup 0139 trial
    and neoadjuvant chemotherapy, 274, 275,
        277, 278
Intrathoracic nodal metastases
    and lymph node dissection, 315–321
    and pulmonary metastasectomy, 315–321

L

Laparoscopy
    and diaphragmatic plication, 338
Lung cancer staging
    EBUS-EUS vs. mediastinoscopy, 243–247
Lung reexpansion
    and diaphragmatic plication, 342
Lymph node accessibility
    and mediastinal staging, 244–246
Lymph node disease
    N1 vs. N2, 320
Lymph node dissection
    and intrathoracic nodal metastases, 315–321
    patient selection for, 321
Lymph node dissection and pulmonary
    metastasectomy, **315–323**
Lymph node metastasis
    and breast carcinoma, 319, 320
    and colorectal carcinoma, 316, 317
    and germ cell tumors, 318, 319
    and head and neck squamous cell carcinoma, 319
    and melanoma, 319
    and nodal status, 320
    and renal cell carcinoma, 317, 318
    and sarcoma, 318

M

Malignant pleural mesothelioma
    extrapleural pneumonectomy for, 360–363
    metaanalysis of, 366–369
    pleurectomy/decortication for, 363–365
    surgery for, 360–372
Management of stage IIIA (N2) non–small cell lung
    cancer, **271–285**
Mediastinal lymphadenectomy
    and survival, 320, 321
Mediastinal staging
    EBUS-EUS vs. mediastinoscopy, 243–247
    endosonography vs. mediastinoscopy, 246
    gold standard for, 244
    in non–small cell lung cancer, 244–247
    patient selection for, 244
    and positron emission tomography, 243, 244
    and video-assisted thoracoscopic surgery, 244,
        245, 247
    vs. surgery, 246
Mediastinal staging: Endosonographic ultrasound
    lymph node biopsy or mediastinoscopy, **243–249**
Mediastinoscopy
    accuracy of, 244–246
    and aortopulmonary window lymph nodes, 247
    complication rate for, 246, 247
    cost of, 247
    and lymph node access, 244–246
    and mediastinal staging, 244–247
    and negative predictive value, 244–246
    and restaging after chemoradiation, 247
    sensitivity of, 244–246
Melanoma
    and lymph node metastasis, 319
    and pulmonary metastasis, 319
Metastases
    in non–small cell lung cancer, 287–292
Metastectomy
    for oligometastatic non–small cell lung cancer,
        287, 291, 292
MPM. See *Malignant pleural mesothelioma.*

N

N2 disease
    management of, 271–282
Neoadjuvant chemotherapy
    and Intergroup 0139 trial, 274, 275, 277, 278
    outcomes of, 279, 280
Non–small cell lung cancer
    adjuvant vs. neoadjuvant chemotherapy, 277, 278
    and conclusions from the literature, 282
    endobronchial ultrasound vs. mediastinoscopy for
        staging, 272

    and evaluation of adjuvant chemotherapy, 278
    evidence-based treatment regimens for, 281
    evolution of multimodality treatment for, 273–275
    and evolving radiation therapy, 281
    and immunotherapy, 281
    and incidentally discovered N2 disease, 277
    management of, 271–282
    and mediastinal staging, 244–247
    and metastasis, 287–292
    and neoadjuvant radiation dose, 279
    and occult N2 disease, 272
    oligometastatic, 287–292
    and persistent N2 disease, 276, 277
    and phase II trials of neoadjuvant chemoradiation,
        274
    pneumonectomy for, 277
    and postoperative radiation therapy, 280, 281
    and proton beam therapy, 281
    and radiation dosage in neoadjuvant setting, 274
    and restaging after neoadjuvant therapy, 272, 273
    staging of, 271–273
    stereotactic body radiation therapy for, 261–268
    and sublobar resection, 251–257
    surgery for, 275–277
    and targeted therapy, 281
    and targeted therapy in stage IIIA regimens, 279
    and tolerance for multimodality treatment
        regimens, 273
    wedge resection vs. segmentectomy, 256
NSCLC. See *Non–small cell lung cancer.*

O

Oligometastatic non–small cell lung cancer
    metastectomy for, 287, 291, 292
    and organ-specific surgical considerations, 289
    principles of surgical treatment for, 288, 289
    and solitary adrenal metastases, 290, 291
    and solitary brain metastasis, 289, 290
    surgery for, 287–292
    and surgical outcomes, 291, 292
Oxibutinin
    for hiperhidrosis, 353

P

P/D. See *Pleurectomy/decortication.*
Palmar hiperhidrosis
    and video-assisted thoracic sympathectomy, 348,
        351, 352
PET. See *Positron emission tomography.*
Plantar hiperhidrosis
    and video-assisted thoracic sympathectomy, 348,
        349, 352
Pleurectomy/decortication

Pleurectomy/decortication (*continued*)
    complications after, 370
    for malignant pleural mesothelioma, 363–365
    and perioperative management, 364
    and postoperative care, 364, 365
    preoperative evaluation for, 363, 364
    results of, 365
    surgical technique for, 364
    vs. extrapleural pneumonectomy, 365–372
Pneumonectomy
    for non–small cell lung cancer, 277
PORT. See *Postoperative radiation therapy.*
Positron emission tomography
    and mediastinal staging, 243, 244
Postoperative radiation therapy
    and non–small cell lung cancer, 280, 281
    trials from the literature, 280
Proton beam therapy
    and non–small cell lung cancer, 281
Pulmonary function tests
    and diaphragmatic paralysis, 334, 335
Pulmonary metastasectomy
    and intrathoracic nodal metastases, 315–321
Pulmonary metastasis
    and breast carcinoma, 319, 320
    and colorectal carcinoma, 316, 317
    and germ cell tumors, 318, 319
    and head and neck squamous cell carcinoma, 319
    and melanoma, 319
    and nodal status, 320
    and renal cell carcinoma, 317, 318
    and sarcoma, 318
Pulmonary toxicity
    and stereotactic body radiation therapy, 266

R

RCC. See *Renal cell carcinoma.*
Renal cell carcinoma
    and lymph node metastasis, 317, 318
    and pulmonary metastasis, 317, 318
Robotic-assisted surgery
    and diaphragmatic plication, 337
The role of induction therapy for esophageal cancer,
    295–304

S

Sarcoma
    and lymph node metastasis, 318
    and pulmonary metastasis, 318
SBRT. See *Stereotactic body radiation therapy.*
SCC. See *Squamous cell carcinoma.*
Squamous cell carcinoma
    of the head and neck, 319
    and lymph node metastasis, 319
    and pulmonary metastasis, 319

Stage IIIA lung cancer
    management of, 271–282
Stent placement for esophageal perforation
    algorithm for, 309
    early implementation of, 306, 307
    exclusion criteria for, 308
    history of, 305, 306
    and hybrid treatment, 306, 307, 312
    outcomes of, 312, 313
    technique for, 308–312
Stereotactic body radiation therapy
    and development of technique, 262
    large database analyses of, 264, 265
    for medically inoperable patients, 262, 263
    for medically operable patients, 263–265
    optimal dose of, 266–268
    in prospective collaborative trials, 262, 263
    in prospective phase II trials, 264
    and pulmonary toxicity, 266
    in randomized phase III trials, 264
    retrospective experience of, 263
    and toxicity, 265, 266
    and toxicity in central tumor locations, 265, 266
    and toxicity in chest wall, 265
    and toxicity in ribs, 265
    and toxicity in skin, 265
Stereotactic body radiation therapy for stage I
    non–small cell lung cancer, **261–269**
Sublobar resection
    and adenocarcinoma, 254, 257
    in elderly patients, 256
    factors effecting outcome of, 255, 256
    and ground glass nodules, 251, 253, 255, 257
    history of, 251, 252
    population-based analysis of, 252
    in prospective randomized trials, 252
    retrospective analysis of, 252–255
    and segmentectomy, 255, 256
    and surgical margin, 255
    and tumor size, 255
Sublobar resection: Ongoing controversy for
    treatment for stage I non–small cell lung cancer,
    251–259
Surgical management of oligometastatic non–small
    cell lung cancer, **287–294**

T

Targeted therapy
    and non–small cell lung cancer, 279, 281
    and thymic tumors, 330, 331
Thymic tumors
    and targeted therapy, 330, 331
    treatment of, 325, 326
Thymoma
    and induction chemoradiation, 328–330
    and induction chemotherapy, 326–328

and induction radiation, 330
and stage IVA disease, 330
Tube thoracostomy
    and diaphragmatic plication, 342

V

VATS. See *Video-assisted thoracic sympathectomy.*
VATS. See *Video-assisted thoracoscopic surgery.*
Video-assisted thoracic sympathectomy
    alternatives to, 352, 353
    anesthesia for, 350
    and azygous lobe, 355
    and chylothorax, 355
    complications of, 355, 356
    contraindications to, 356
    failure of, 356, 357
    and functional reorganization, 357
    and hemorrhage, 355
    for hiperhidrosis, 347–357

and Horner syndrome, 356
and incomplete surgery, 356
instruments for, 350
and paresis, 356
and paresthesia, 356
patient positioning for, 350
and pleural adherences, 355
and pneumothorax, 355
and postoperative pain, 356
and pulmonary atelectasis, 355
and regeneration, 357
results of, 354, 355
and subcutaneous emphysema, 355
technique for, 350, 351
and transitory brachycardia, 356
Video-assisted thoracic sympathectomy for
    hyperhidrosis, **347–358**
Video-assisted thoracoscopic surgery
    and diaphragmatic plication, 337
    and mediastinal staging, 244, 245, 247

Moving?

Make sure your subscription moves with you!

To notify us of your new address, find your **Clinics Account Number** (located on your mailing label above your name), and contact customer service at:

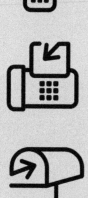

Email: journalscustomerservice-usa@elsevier.com

800-654-2452 (subscribers in the U.S. & Canada)
314-447-8871 (subscribers outside of the U.S. & Canada)

Fax number: 314-447-8029

Elsevier Health Sciences Division
Subscription Customer Service
3251 Riverport Lane
Maryland Heights, MO 63043

Printed and bound by CPI Group (UK) Ltd, Croydon, CR0 4YY

08/05/2025

01864686-0013